"Colette Bouchez has taken all the skills you'd expect from an award-winning journalist and mixed them with a big dose of the latest information in order to attack an area of Women's Health that has previously been woefully neglected. Good for her!"—Steven R. Goldstein, M.D., Professor of Obstetrics and Gynecology, New York University School of Medicine, and author of *Could It Be . . . Perimenopause?*

"*The V Zone* offers clear and comprehensive explanations for the prevention and treatment of gynecologic diseases. Colette Bouchez's concise style is a pleasure to read. I especially enjoyed, and learned from, the 'Q&A' and 'An Expert's Opinion On' sections in each chapter. *The V Zone* is now in our Resource Center Library."—Alison Estabrook, M.D., Chief, Breast Surgery, St. Luke's–Roosevelt Hospital Center, and Professor of Clinical Surgery, Columbia University

"A book that helps every woman to not only know and understand her body better, but to learn how to better communicate with her doctor in a way that is bound to have a positive impact on her life-long health care."—Reginald Puckett, M.D., OB/GYN, New York Hospital–Cornell Medical Center

"Finally! A resource guide women can not only understand, but really trust to help them quickly and easily identify even their most intimate health problems, and then find the best treatment options available. It's like a Sunday afternoon chat with a *really* smart girlfriend—about a subject that's been neglected for far too long!" —Tina Mosetis, formerly Director of Communications, American Cancer Society of New York City

"Move over, *Our Bodies, Ourselves*—Colette Bouchez's *The V Zone* is the one essential guide every woman needs on her bookshelf. The best part—Bouchez cuts through all the doctorspeak and puts the power of diagnosis, prevention and even cure back into the patient's hands. And does it without the smug snobbery of most medical books, which visit upon readers either the high-minded (and mostly incomprehensible) jargon of the hospital room or the touchy-feely soft focus of the alternative mindset. Bouchez, in a straightforward and surprisingly witty star turn, distills all the best of modern, ancient and folk medicine into a clear and compelling guide."—Shirley Mathews, Managing Editor, HealthScout.com

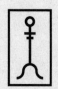

Colette Bouchez

With a Foreword by
Elsa-Grace V. Giardina, M.D., Director,
THE CENTER FOR WOMEN'S HEALTH,
Columbia Presbyterian Medical Center

A FIRESIDE BOOK
Published by Simon & Schuster
New York London Toronto Sydney Singapore

THE V

ZONE

A Woman's Guide to Intimate Health Care

FIRESIDE
Rockefeller Center
1230 Avenue of the Americas
New York, NY 10020

Copyright © 2001 Colette Bouchez
All rights reserved,
including the right of reproduction
in whole or in part in any form.

FIRESIDE and colophon are registered trademarks
of Simon & Schuster, Inc.

Designed by Bonni Leon-Berman

Manufactured in the United States of America

3 5 7 9 10 8 6 4 2

Library of Congress Cataloging-in-Publication Data

Bouchez, Colette.
 The V zone : a woman's guide to intimate health care / Colette Bouchéz ; with a
foreword by Elsa-Grace V. Giardina.
  p. cm.
 1. Women—Health and hygiene. 2. Gynecology. I. Title.

RG121.B75 2001
618.1—dc21   2001018152

ISBN 0-684-87097-5 (trade pbk.)

ACKNOWLEDGMENTS

My deepest gratitude goes to the hundreds of physicians and medical researchers who have toiled long and hard to focus our attention on the importance of women's health care. I am forever indebted to their dedication and am proud that their efforts and their words ring loud and clear throughout the pages of this book. My admiration is particularly profound for the physicians, nurses, and other health professionals at the Women's Center at Columbia Presbyterian Medical Center and the Women's Health Center at New York-Presbyterian Weill Cornell Medical Center, whose efforts on behalf of women have never faltered.

My sincere thanks go to Dr. Elsa-Grace V. Giardina, director of the Center for Women's Health at Columbia Presbyterian Medical Center, for her kind words and her friendship. You are a guiding light for us all.

I owe a huge debt of gratitude to former Simon & Schuster editor Betsy Radin Herman, whose sparks of creativity stirred my own passions for women's health and helped me create the framework for this book. Her inspiration and her friendship have been a gift from heaven.

And to the "adopted" mommy of this project, editor Marcela Landres, I can only say, "Thank you, thank you, thank you." You picked up all the pieces and put them all in the right places, and you smiled through it all. As an editor, you are a writer's best friend, and I could not have done this without you. You are a true treasure!

Another to whom I owe more than words can say is editor Eleanor Rawson, the true grande dame of publishing and the woman who made it possible for all the rest of us to break through the glass ceilings. Thank you for mapping the road ahead, and especially for teaching me not only how to write a book but how to be a writer.

Thanks to my gal pals in the newsroom—Barbara, Tracey, Rosemary, Emily, Edna-Jean, and especially Tina. Your laughter kept me going, and you won't have to listen hard to hear your voices through-out this book.

Special thanks to my dear and special friend Bill Fichter, manager of Trump Palace, and his entire staff, particularly Tom, John, Tommy, Chris, Johnny, Danny, Fernando, Mark, Nazmi, Joe, and Kevin. Your kindness, loyalty, and friendship will always be remembered.

A special thank you also goes out to Susan Parker, former director of public affairs for Columbia Presbyterian Medical Center. Undoubtedly she was always a journalist's best friend. Thanks also go to Myrna Manners, Kathleen Robinson, and Jonathan Weill of New York-Presbyterian Hospital, Weill Cornell Medical Center, and Columbia Presbyterian Medical Center Department of Public Affairs for always having all the right answers and all the right experts. And special thanks to Peter Ferrara and Lynn Odell of New York University Medical Center for always guiding me to the very best medical opinions.

Most assuredly, I owe an enormous debt of gratitude to Fireside publisher Mark Gompertz for taking a chance on this book, and particularly to editor-in-chief Trish Todd, who believed not only in this project but in my ability to make it happen. It is a privilege and an honor to be on your team.

To St. Jude: Thank you for everything and for always being there to pull me through.

Finally, a very heartfelt thank you to my dear friend Dr. Niels H. Lauersen, a physician and healer who has taught me more about medicine and life than I could ever say. His work to further the cause of women's health care has been the inspiration behind all of my own efforts, and his voice, his wisdom, and, most profoundly, his spirit soar through every page of this book.

To my mother,
who gave me everything and whose love
will be forever in my heart,
and to my dad—the memory of him is my gift from God.

And to all the smart, strong, and wonderful women in my family:
Grandma Ann, Helen, Mid, Dee, BettyAnn, Patty, Annie,
Bonnie, Cindy, Andrea, Suzanne, Maria, Laurie, and Michelle,
and all our daughters and grandaughters:
Thank you for sharing your courage, your love,
and your passion for life.
You are my heroes.
And to NHL—you will always be the
wind beneath my wings.

CONTENTS

CONTENTS

FOREWORD

It wasn't so very long ago that most of what we knew about a woman's body we learned from studying men.

Because women were virtually excluded from most major medical studies, doctors were forced simply to extrapolate what we learned about the male body and apply it to the female body. While sometimes this line of thinking worked—and the knowledge could be applied to both sexes—more often than not, we came up short. Indeed, sometimes it seemed as if the more we learned about men, the more we realized how little we knew about women. And nowhere was our lack of knowledge more obvious than in the area of intimate health.

From simple vaginal bacteria and annoying yeast infections, to more complex and potentially serious problems like pelvic inflammatory disease and sexually transmitted diseases, to life-threatening conditions like cancer, heart disease, and stroke, the lack of research was astounding. In many instances we did not even have the necessary tools to diagnose some of these problems properly, let alone take steps to prevent them from occurring.

Fortunately, things are changing—and quite dramatically. In the past decade, and particularly in the past five years, women's health issues finally began to attract the attention they have long deserved. As a physician, I am pleased to report that gender science is taking a more prominent position in key research agendas the world over. Thanks in part to a new women's research initiative sponsored by the National Institutes of Health (NIH), as well as the establishment of the Office of Research on Women's Health and federal changes in NIH guidelines, not only are women now being included in major medical studies of all kinds, they are also getting a fair share of research devoted exclusively to "female health problems." Indeed, we have learned more in the past decade about how a woman's body functions—and what causes it to malfunction—than we ever dreamed. For you, that means not only the opportunity for more comprehensive medical care, but also the chance to maintain your good health longer.

As encouraging as all this has been, however, statistics continue to remind us just how far we still have to go. As I write to you, the AIDS epidemic among women continues to rise, heart disease and stroke remain major killers, and female cancers continue to claim lives. Smoking and its consequence, lung cancer, are rising faster and are more deadly than even breast cancer; and infertility plagues us in record numbers, as vaginal infections and even sexually transmitted diseases go undiagnosed and untreated, often until irreversible damage occurs.

Why is this happening? Unfortunately, there are many women who do not take full advantage of all medical science has to offer.

For some, it's all about a simple lack of recognition of risk factors. Too many times I find patients who, despite what they see and hear in the news every day, continue to overlook their own personal vulnerability to a wide variety of intimate health concerns. For others, it is simply the outdated taboos surrounding these subjects that keep them in the dark. Indeed, for many women, it remains difficult or impossible even to broach certain intimate care issues, let alone seek treatment, even in the safe and trusting confines of their doctor's office. And for still others, it is a lack of access to truly comprehensive medical treatment. Unfortunately, if you don't know what kind of care you *should* be getting, it's difficult to judge the quality of the care you *are* receiving.

The important news is that it doesn't have to be this way. The knowledge and the expertise are there—if you know where to find it. Which is why I am especially delighted to introduce you to *The V Zone,* a book that I believe will help every woman take full advantage of what medicine today has to offer.

Indeed, not only will it empower you with the knowledge you need right now to achieve the best health care possible, it will also help you take full advantage of prevention strategies, ensuring that you maintain good health in the future. Equally vital, this is a book that will help foster a more open and ultimately a healthier relationship between you and your doctor—and in doing so ensure you continue to maintain optimum medical care for the rest of your life.

Perhaps most important of all, *The V Zone* is not just a new book. It's a *new attitude,* one that dismisses taboos linked to intimate health in ways that allow you to know, understand, and even appreciate your body in a whole new way. If you are a mother, I urge you to share what you discover in this book with your daughter. If you are a daughter, talk to your mother, your best friend, and your sisters about what you learn here.

Indeed, it is only when we break down the barriers to communication within our own gender and share what we know that we can begin to achieve true equality in our health care and in our lives.

The medical profession is catching up with the importance of women's health issues. Now it's up to you to make the best use of what we have learned—and how far we have come. I hope you enjoy your journey through *The V Zone* and that you will be as enlightened and enthusiastic about the future of your good health as I am.

Elsa-Grace V. Giardina, M.D.
Professor of Clinical Medicine
Director, The Center for Women's Health
Columbia Presbyterian Medical Center, Columbia University
New York City

PREFACE

It's Your Body—And It's Your Life

When I began my journalism career in the early 1980s, one of my first medical interviews was with the renowned obstetrician-gynecologist Niels H. Lauersen. At the time, Dr. Lauersen had just coined the phrase "It's Your Body" (also the title of his landmark book), and it came to represent a vital aspect of the women's movement: the importance of taking responsibility for your own health.

Indeed, as the revolution pressed forward, bit by bit we all began to see that women no longer were destined to remain silently under the controlling power of a male-dominated medical profession, with little or nothing to say about the quality of care we would receive. Instead, we were being urged to learn about our *own* body and to participate in our health care decisions—and ultimately to find the kind of doctor who would allow us to develop an equal partnership of nurturing care.

I am an investigative medical writer, and this philosophy hit home in a way nothing else ever had before. Not only did it verify a concept I had always believed—the importance of being an aggressive and savvy health consumer—but it also validated one of the professional goals I had set for myself a long time before: I would do everything I could to make certain that all women had equal access to the kind of straightforward, "grown-up" medical information *necessary* to take control of not only their health care but their lives.

It is a concept and an ideal that I am convinced holds even greater importance for women today. As we enter into this new millennium, we enter into a time when all too often managed care, not medical care, is the deciding factor between sickness and health—and sometimes even life and death. For many of us, it will be the ability to rally our own personal medical agenda that ensures we receive any care at all.

Nowhere is this truer than in the area of our intimate health. For many women it is in fact the V zone (that sacred, revered, and some-times feared area that lies quietly between our belly button and our thighs) which will represent some of the greatest health challenges. From potentially devastating problems like endometriosis, ovarian cysts, fibroid tumors, pelvic inflammatory disease, reproductive can-cers, and a slew of sexually transmitted viruses and infections, to everyday concerns like vaginitis, yeast infections, and urinary tract infections, a woman's intimate geography is such that few among us can ever completely avoid at least some of these problems.

The reassuring news here is that in most instances, simple knowl-edge about our body may be all that's necessary to offset the risk of even potentially deadly V zone disease.

The bad news is that the kind of intimate body awareness necessary to accomplish this often does not come easy. Why? Beginning as early as childhood, the vagina seemed destined to remain cloaked in a veil of secrecy, hidden even from our own wondering curiosity. While lit-tle boys were continually urged to explore their bodies and applauded for learning to handle their genitals with deft and ease, little girls were given the opposite message. "Don't look—and don't even think about touching yourself" was the mantra that followed many of us right into adulthood. And in many ways that mind-set has affected our health and our health care in a very negative way. Life-saving breast exams, for example, are to this day met with great resistance among the gen-eral female population, ostensibly because of antiquated ideas about touching ourselves. The vulvar self-exam, now considered by many doctors to be an essential part of preventative self-care, is meeting with even greater resistance for pretty much the same reasons. Indeed, when it comes to protecting and preserving our V zone health, a num-ber of taboo attitudes are keeping women from not only achieving op-timum intimate health but also optimum health care.

But our own attitudes about V zone health are only part of the stumbling block to getting the care we deserve and need. Indeed, in many instances, the medical profession itself is also to blame. Cer-tainly there are many fine gynecologists throughout the nation, many of whom not only appreciate a well-educated patient but do every-thing they can to encourage women to learn about their bodies and take the important initiative in their own health care. Not coincidentally, these are usually the same physicians who also remain at the forefront of the latest research, treatment, and care.

All too often, however, there are just as many doctors who are getting away with offering women less than optimum attention.

In some instances, it is the doctor's own ignorance about the latest research that is to blame. By not taking the time to keep up with the latest treatment options, they are unable to offer their patients all they deserve.

In other instances, it is the health care system itself that is to blame. Indeed, even today, too many women's health care issues remain at the bottom of the research agenda. Thus, without all the noise generated by big money, headline studies, often the small but significant advances that *are* made on behalf of women remain vastly underreported. Even the most well-meaning physicians can overlook important results—facts and factors that for you could make an important difference in the quality of care you receive. In some instances, it could even mean the difference between quick, efficient care and undue suffering, or even fatal complications.

And too, sadly, we cannot overlook the limitations placed on the medical profession itself by managed care, as well as many independent insurance companies—both of which can tie the hands of even the best doctors, keeping them from giving you the best care possible. Whether it be restrictions in time (such as appointments that are too short to cover all the bases) or limitations in treatment options covered by various medical plans, the level of your personal health care can become so restricted that unless you know what you are missing, you will have little chance of making a case to get what you deserve.

Finally, we cannot overlook the unfortunate truth that even in these politically correct and enlightened times, women still suffer a good deal of what I call "medical chauvinism." Even doctors who purportedly dedicate their lives to caring for female patients can do so in a way that is so condescending that it subjects us all to still another level of substandard care. As our problems and our complaints are dismissed with a gratuitous pat on the head and the suggestion to "leave the worrying to me," we are being left in the dark about not only what is wrong but all that can done to fix it.

If all this sounds a little pessimistic and even somewhat depressing,

I'm here to tell you there is definitely a silver lining in this cloud. Indeed, overcoming these obstacles and changing the face of women's intimate health care can be accomplished—*one woman at a time*—and it can begin with you. With very little effort and just a few key pieces of knowledge, you can take the steps necessary not only to ensure your own intimate health care, under any and all circumstances, but in doing so also contribute to the larger tapestry of better care for us all.

For all these reasons, I have chosen to write this book—one that I hope will break down the barriers and leave behind the taboos associated with intimate health care, and as it does also guide you safely and securely to the most important and necessary steps you can take to get the best possible V zone health care, now and in the future. As a medical reporter for a major urban newspaper for nearly two decades, I have employed the sum of my investigative experience to bring you up to date on not only the kinds of intimate health problems you are facing today but also the latest diagnostic and treatment options available to help. And I have done all I can to show you how to use this knowledge to work with your doctor, ensuring the best intimate health care possible.

Here is just some of what you will find in this book:

- the new vagina virus—and how it can affect your sex life
- the new bacterial vaginitis—and how to keep it from harming your fertility
- understanding painful sex—and the latest treatments that can help
- recurring urinary tract infections (UTIs)—and why research shows you don't have to suffer anymore
- the yeast infection treatment maze—how to get out alive and healthy
- women and AIDS—with information you can't afford to ignore
- the latest in Pap smear technologies—and what your doctor should be doing to protect your V zone health and maybe save your life
- the sexually transmitted cancer—and how to protect yourself

And that's just the beginning!

Because I have always been a strong advocate of natural health care, *The V Zone* also offers you something you may not find in other books: natural solutions to many V zone problems. Indeed, featured throughout the book are special sections titled "Mother Nature's Bounty," each offering one or more self-care options based on *scientifically researched* and in many instances medically proven ways of using natural medicine to treat V zone health concerns.

Another one of my areas of interest and concern is intimate hygiene, particularly in regard to the items we all use in everyday life— from menstrual products like tampons and sanitary pads, to douches, sprays, deodorants, powders, even the "condiments" of our sex life like lubricants, foams, jellies, and condoms. Although a good many of these products are safe and effective, research has shown that too many of these items carry health risks, many of which have been kept from women for way too long. Indeed, during my nearly fifteen years as a medical writer for *The New York Daily News,* I was proud and happy to bring some of these issues to public light, many of them for the first time. As a result of several of my investigative reports, local and federal legislation was launched that, when passed, will vastly improve the safety of many women's intimate health care products and make self-care even more effective for us all. Later in this book you will learn about everything that I have uncovered—and the steps you can take right now to help ensure the safety of the products you do use.

Because no one can write a truly comprehensive medical book without relying on the opinions of experts in each given field, I am happy to report that in this book you will find some of the best of those opinions. Indeed, despite all the problems in women's health care, there are in fact many wonderful doctors who not only share our concerns but whose research and expertise have helped form and expand the base of our health care knowledge in many important ways. Throughout this book you will find what I believe are some of the most progressive and important viewpoints about a wide variety of V zone topics, including some you may have been unable to discuss with your own doctor.

I hope you will also take a few moments to read through the special resources section at the end of the book. Not only will it provide you with the tools you need to find even more in-depth information about the subjects covered in this book, but it will also give you a jump-start on getting the best health care possible via a contact list of the National Centers for Excellence in Women's Health Care. Indeed, some seventeen medical centers around the nation have been designated by the National Institutes of Health as providing women with the optimum in medical care. If you are not satisfied with your health practitioner or if you are seeking a second opinion about the care you are receiving, I urge you to make use of these centers, to contact their doctors and when possible to visit the various hospitals and institutions that have worked hard to put women's health at the top of their priority list.

In addition, I also invite you to turn to "Resources for Better Health" for information on how to contact the American Medical Women's Association (AMWA), a nationwide organization of female physicians dedicated to fostering the highest standards in women's health care. In 1999 I was privileged to be one of only a few journalists to become a member of the AMWA, which, much like the American Medical Association (AMA) is there to help both doctors and patients alike in the pursuit of the best medical care possible. The AMWA's vast network of medical specialists can help you locate a physician in your area who will honor and appreciate the fact that you are taking responsibility for your health, and who will work with you in a partnership of preventative care.

As I close this Preface and invite you to begin your journey of intimate exploration, I would like to leave you with this one final thought: After all is said and done, don't ever forget that it *is* your body, and it is *your* life—and only you can take the steps necessary to ensure that you remain healthy and strong throughout all of your days.

If I can ever help you to do that in any way, please write to me—and do send any questions you may have about the information in this book, or about any aspect of your health. To do so, visit me on the Web at www.TheVzone.net. Here you can not only post your questions, but also find the very latest updates on all aspects of women's health.

My Warmest Regards,
Colette Bouchez

CHAPTER ONE

Understanding Your V Zone

What You Need to Know About Your Intimate Health

If you're like most other women, it's likely you pay very little attention to your intimate anatomy until a problem occurs. Then you panic, as you begin to realize how little you really know about some areas of your body. Indeed, studies show that, by and large, *most* of us are far more familiar with the pores on our nose than we are with our V zone, the area between our belly button and our thighs. And that can be a big mistake.

Why? First, the more you know about your intimate anatomy, the greater is your chance of having not only a happier and more satisfying sex life but, more important, a healthier one, for you and your partner.

More important, *not* being familiar with how this area of your body functions can have some dire consequences. Indeed, the placement and structure of a woman's intimate geography is such that each of us is at risk for a variety of diseases and conditions, several of which carry some potentially serious complications. If you're not familiar with what's normal for you, then you may have a real problem figuring out when something goes wrong—at least early enough to get the kind of comprehensive treatment that offsets the risk of any of those serious health consequences from occurring.

What's that you say? You're counting on your doctor to provide you with all the V zone protection you need? Then you may be surprised to learn studies have shown that your gynecologist may not be offering you the care you deserve. Indeed, at least one new report, a 1999 survey of doctors conducted by the National Vaginitis Association, revealed that the majority of gynecologists sometimes bypass offering patients treatment for even potentially serious vaginal infections unless they themselves bring symptoms to their doctor's attention. *And this can be the case even when the doctor notices problems during the exam.* Perhaps the worst part is that the doctors surveyed didn't even provide a reason. *They simply said they don't do it!*

Indeed, if you are to be ensured the best, most progressive, most preventative health care possible, you must become an active participant in that health care. And ultimately that means knowing enough about your body to enable you to recognize when something *does* go wrong.

When it comes to learning about your V zone, the best place to start is with a little healthy self-exploration, done with a keen eye toward becoming familiar with form *and* function. In short, you need to know not only how your intimate anatomy looks and feels under normal conditions of optimum health, but also how it acts and reacts.

With that goal in mind, this book begins with a kind of personal road map—a "geography," if you will—of a woman's most intimate parts, with emphasis on helping you learn more about what's normal for you—*and* what's not.

If you already believe you know more about your body than you probably will ever need to, feel free to skim this chapter and proceed to the areas of the book that apply to your V zone health needs right now.

But if you're not really sure about how much you do or don't know, then I invite you to pay special attention to this chapter. If, in fact, you take only one message from this book, let it be that you can have power over your body and your health care—once you take the time to get to know yourself.

Your V Zone Road Map: Where to Begin

Your journey of self-exploration starts with the area just below your "bikini line"—the area of your V zone known as the *vulva*. For most of us, the portion we are most familiar with is the *mons veneris,* or *mound of Venus,* a wad of fatty tissue that lies just on top of the opening to the vagina. Usually covered with pubic hair, it acts as a protective cover particularly during vigorous intercourse, helping to absorb impact and sheltering the more delicate organs and bones in and around the pelvis. Not coincidentally, this section of your V zone is also among the most erotic areas of your body, highly sensitive to the touch. In fact, the pubic hair found here can be *so* responsive that even a light touch can cause a sensual, electric-like shock sensation that travels right to the inside of your vagina.

Following the mound of Venus downward, you will come to the *labia majora,* or outside vaginal lips. Also made up of pads of fatty tissue covered with pubic hair, these "lips" are also extremely sensitive to both touch and temperature. In fact, much like a man's testicles, which shrink and wrinkle in response to cold temperatures, so do a woman's labia. They also swell and become puffy and softer in warmer temperatures, particularly when you are bathing in a hot tub or sauna or when you are sexually aroused. For some women, simply stroking the outside of the labia majora can act as powerful foreplay.

Inside the labia majora is a second set of "lips," known as the *labia minora.* Composed of a thin tissue with an elastic quality, they work to protect the interior of your vagina. In some women the labia minora are hardly visible; in others they are large and protruding. Both types, and anything in between, are considered normal.

Although most often we think of our intimate secretions and discharges as coming from the vagina, in fact, most come from the walls lining the outside and inside of the outer vulvar lips. Both the labia majora and labia minora contain an abundance of sweat, scent, and oil glands that continuously secrete the fluids that keep the vagina moist and healthy and provide the characteristic musky scent and extra "wet" sensation when you are sexually aroused. These secretions also help protect the vagina from acids and other irritating chemicals in urine and menstrual blood, as well as help block the passage of some bacteria into the reproductive tract.

Nestled neatly into the folds of the labia is your actual vagina. Although it is only about ¾ of an inch wide and extends just 3 to 4 inches inward, it is composed of highly elastic tissue and stretches dramatically to many times its original size. This makes it possible not only to give birth but also to comfortably accommodate a penis of virtually any size. To help make intercourse easier and more pleasurable for both sexes, the inside of the vagina also has a pleated-like surface called *rugae*. Similar to the folds found in corrugated cardboard, the rugae help grip the penis and ease it deeper inside. After intercourse, as well as childbirth, your vagina contracts back to its normal size.

Located deeper inside the vagina is the *hymen*, a thin membrane that in the not too distant past was thought to function as a kind of archaic "virginity meter." As the myth went, on first intercourse the hymen would tear, causing bleeding to occur. If that characteristic bloodshed didn't take place, a woman's virginity was put into question. Today we know just how foolish (if not insulting) this myth really is. Indeed, so many factors can cause the hymen to tear, including most sporting activities, that even a doctor can't tell if a woman is a virgin simply by looking to this membrane for clues.

Although its shape and size is as individual as the woman herself (hymens can range from a thin, wispy membrane to a tough, fibrous layer), in some women it can be so thick that it won't break even during sex, which can cause any attempt at intercourse to be extremely painful. In fact, if you have always experienced pain or discomfort during intercourse, one of the first areas your doctor should check is your hymen. Should it be exceptionally thick, your gynecologist can remove it by a relatively fast and simple in-office procedure.

SEX AND YOUR VAGINA

Your entire vaginal canal, as well as your labia majora and minora are covered in sensitive nerve endings capable of responding to touch and stimulation. For many women, however, the "command central" of sexual responsiveness is the clitoris. This tiny organ, composed of soft, spongy tissue and covered by a hood of skin (called the *prepuce*), sits atop the inner folds of your vagina, a scant ¾ of an inch in length. Once you are sexually stimulated, the hood pulls back. Then, much like a penis, the clitoris begins filling with blood, which more than doubles its size, and it becomes firm, erect, and highly sensitive to the touch. Indeed, although it remains a lot smaller than a penis, the clitoris contains the exact same number of nerve endings—which is one reason that its erotic effect can seem so intense. If for any reason this clitoral activity does not take place (for example, if there is a congenital defect), an orgasm may not be possible.

In addition, many women find intense sexual pleasure from an area of the vagina known as the *G spot*. Some contend that it is only a myth, but for those who claim to have experienced its ecstasy, it is said to be a powerhouse of sexual stimulation. If you're seeking to find your personal G spot, look approximately one-third to one-half way into your vagina (see illustration). If you think you have found it, use two fingers and add a little pressure. If it's there, you'll know it!

More V Zone Anatomy: What Else You Need to Know

In addition to your vulva, your intimate anatomy also involves the following areas:

Urethra—Located just below your clitoris, this is the passageway for urine. About 3 inches long, it extends inward and is connected to your bladder. Containing mucus-secreting glands, it also helps pro-

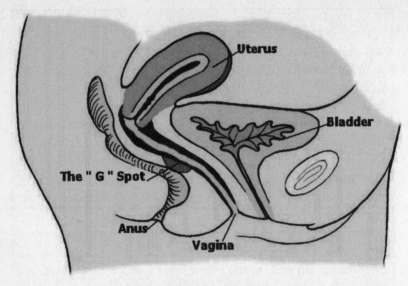

THE G SPOT

Although its existence is hotly debated, those who believe in the infamous
G spot of sexual excitement say it is located between the vagina and the anus
and can be reached by going one-third to one-half way into the vaginal canal.
Courtesy of Lippincott, Williams & Wilkins, Medi-Clip

duce a fluid that keeps your bladder opening moist and less likely to
become irritated.

Perineum—A short piece of skin that stretches from the bottom of
the vagina to the anal opening. Because the perineum can tear during
childbirth, some obstetricians recommend cutting the skin just before the baby is ready to leave the birth channel. This, however, is
considered controversial, and not all physicians agree it's necessary.

Bartholin's glands—Located on either side of the vaginal opening,
these tiny glands produce small amounts of lubricating fluid, particularly during sex. Sometimes these glands can become inflamed,
causing pain and swelling and, ultimately, infection (see Chapter 4).

Cervix—Located at the end of the vagina and composed of smooth
muscle and collagen fibers, the cervix acts as the gateway to the

uterus. Its size can range from 1 to 3 millimeters (between 0.04 and 0.12 inches), changing in response to various stages of a single menstrual cycle. Although it is technically part of the vagina, the cells lining the inside of the cervix look and grow differently, making them much more susceptible to infection.

Uterus—Shaped much like a small pear and about the same size, the uterus is the main organ of your entire reproductive system (see illustration). It is lined with layers of cells, one of which responds to hormonal stimulation. This stimulation causes the lining to grow thick during each menstrual cycle and be shed in the form of menstrual blood each month. Should pregnancy occur, the lining becomes the spongy nest where your fertilized egg implants and where your baby grows and develops.

Ovaries—Attached to the uterus by strong but thin ligaments are the ovaries, the main producers of the primary female hormone estrogen. In addition, the ovaries also play host to some 400,000 egg follicles—

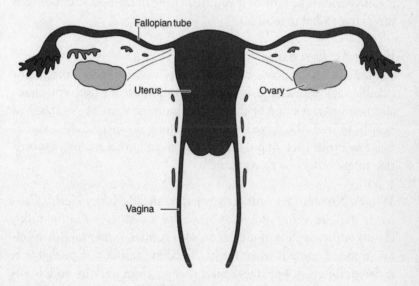

A WOMAN'S REPRODUCTIVE SYSTEM

or "fertility seeds"—one of which develops into a fertile egg and is ovulated, usually every month during the childbearing years.

Fallopian tubes—Just 3 to 4 inches in length and a delicate ⅓ of an inch in diameter, these slender tubes jut out from either side of the uterus and slope gently downward toward the ovary. The finger-like ends, which resemble the open petals of a flower, reach out to catch an ovulated egg. The fallopian tubes also act as the transport lane for sperm, which swim toward the egg in anticipation of fertilization. If fertilization does occur, tiny hairs (called *cilia*), which line the inside of the tube, help shuttle the fertilized egg into the uterus, where it can implant and begin to grow.

Your Healthy Body: Know the Signs

When it comes to a healthy V zone, there are three major factors to look for. They include the way your vulva looks and feels to the touch, how it smells, and the quality of your intimate secretions or discharge. All three factors, alone or together, can help you determine if your V zone is healthy or if you are in need of medical attention and care. Here's what to look for.

Factor #1: Discharge

Medically known as *leukorrhea,* many women believe that a noticeable vaginal discharge is always an indication of a problem. In reality, however, it's one of the most important signs of *good* vaginal health. Indeed, the vagina is a self-cleaning organ, and discharge is one way it rids itself of old cells, bacteria, and other microorganisms that might otherwise cause harm.

What's Normal: According to experts at the McKinley Health Center at the University of Illinois, look for a discharge that is milky, cloudy white, or clear. If it dries on your panties, it may take on a yellow tinge or contain white flecks. Since the amount of discharge is different for every woman—and it changes from week to week in direct response to the menstrual cycle—it's difficult to say what's normal in this respect. That said, for the most part, discharge should be visible but not so abundant as to make you feel you are wetting your panties all day long. You should know, however, that stress can affect vaginal discharge (increasing or decreasing it), as can birth control pills. Sexual arousal will almost always increase production (that's normal!), while just after pregnancy and during breast-feeding, discharge often decreases, making your vagina feel somewhat drier.

Red Flags: Problems include discharge that appears grayish-white or yellow-green in color; is clumpy or "cheesy" looking; a frothy or foaming discharge of any color; and exceptional amounts of discharge, particularly if it is runny, watery, or very thin.

What This Means to You: For the large majority of women these particular red flags usually signal the presence of any number of simple vaginal infections—and you'll learn more about what they are and how they are treated later in this book. In a few rare instances, however, they could signal the presence of more complicated and serious problems, including pelvic inflammatory disease or even cancer. However, as with all other medical problems, the faster you are diagnosed, the more likely it is that you will suffer no permanent consequences. So don't panic—but don't avoid seeing your doctor.

Factor #2: Vaginal Odors

Every woman has a personal intimate scent unique to her, and it's generally magnified during sexual arousal as well as during ovulation and sometimes menstruation. In fact, some studies have shown that it is this natural scent of "reproduction" that throws a man back to his most primal mating instincts, causing him to feel more "turned on" to a woman when she is the most fertile.

What's Normal: Under healthy circumstances, a vagina should have no offensive odor—but that doesn't mean you won't smell *something*. In addition to your personal biochemical scent, most healthy women will also notice a faint salty or slightly musky odor.

Red Flags: Look for a "fishy" or foul odor—sometimes described as a bitter or sour smell. Also note any pungent smell that seems obvi-

THE MENSTRUAL CYCLE AND VAGINAL DISCHARGE

Although a variety of infections and vaginal disorders can change the color, consistency, or amount of discharge, perhaps the factor that makes the most difference on a regular basis is your menstrual cycle. Here's what to expect:

• Beginning of cycle (days 1 through 12): After bleeding stops, discharge is at a minimum and milky white in color. As you approach the middle of your cycle, it will begin to flow more copiously and may look clearer.

• Just prior to ovulation (days 12 to 14): Discharge is abundant and takes on a clear, more liquid appearance—something that causes some women to feel "wet" during this time.

• After ovulation (days 14 to 28): Discharge is whiter in appearance and more opaque. Since it contains more cervical mucus, it will also be thicker in consistency.

ous, such as overly salty or oily, or any disturbing odors that appear directly after intercourse. All can signal the beginnings of a vaginal infection. Also be on the lookout for what can only be described as a vague smell of freshly baked bread. It could signal a yeast infection. At the same time, remember that what may *seem* like an intimate odor could actually be coming from an area outside the vagina, such as the groin, where many women tend to sweat profusely during warm weather. In addition, certain foods can change the scent of your urine (sometimes making it smell stronger or more ammonia-like), which may make it seem as if your vagina is emanating an odor when it's not. These smells do not indicate a vaginal problem and should not be confused with true, intimate odors.

What This Means to You: Most often a vaginal odor that does not disappear with good hygiene is usually the sign of some type of infection. (You'll learn more about what those infections are in upcoming chapters.) In the meantime, you should also check the presence of any accompanying discharge (see Factor #1 above), as this can help narrow down the possible causes of the odor itself.

But with or without discharge, do bring the odor to your doctor's attention. *Important note:* When you see your doctor (and all abnormal odors and discharges should be checked firsthand and not diagnosed over the telephone), do not attempt to cover up the smell by using a scented body wash or talc before your visit. Instead, wash with plain, warm water and dry well. Remember, you *want* your doctor to smell what you smell.

Factor #3: Genital Skin Condition and Color

Sometimes the earliest signs of V zone infection are indicated by how your vulva looks and feels, particularly in regard to itching or significant changes in texture or color.

What's Normal: The area on the inside and the outside of your vagina should be smooth, free of bumps, dark or light spots, blisters, or rashes. The color on the inside of the outer lips should be a fairly uniform shade of light pink, or, in women of color, a slightly darker, salmon-color pink. The deeper inside you go, the darker the skin looks, up to a medium red.

You should also check the area just outside your vagina, particularly at your panty line, where your thighs meet your groin. It should be free of any swelling as well as bumps or lumps.

Red Flags: Look for bumps; rashes; redness; itching; lumps; lesions; white or light patches, particularly inside the vulva; dark patches or areas of very red or reddish-purple tissue; areas that burn or are painful to the touch; and significant changes in pubic hair, such as obvious thinning.

What This Means to You: For most women, these red flags are usually the result of simple dermatological-type problems, often caused by any number of environmental factors such as the fabric or style of your panties or even your laundry detergent (see Chapter 4). In a few instances these same symptoms could also be the sign of minor infection or even a biochemical imbalance such as a thyroid disorder—

and even more rarely, a more complicated disease such as genital warts or even rare forms of cancer. The key here is not to try to diagnose these problems yourself. Later in this book you will learn more about how and why many of these conditions develop. Use that information to open a dialogue with your doctor—and be certain always to mention any changes in genital skin, color, and condition during your exam.

The V Zone Self-Exam

Now that you're familiar with how your V zone *should* function during optimal health, it's time to find out if indeed it *is* functioning this way now. The best way to tell that is by some self-exploration, in the form of a vulvar self-exam. Indeed, experts advise that checking yourself on a regular basis (some say as often as you do a monthly breast exam) is one of the best ways to catch most health problems *before* they go on to become catastrophic problems.

Getting Started

To begin your exam you need only two things: a hand mirror and a good source of light. According to the Center for Vulvar Disease, before every exam be certain to wash your hands thoroughly, lathering with soap for 15 to 20 seconds and then rinsing in warm water. Since you will be touching the inside of your body, it is imperative that you don't skip this important step.

That done, you must position your body in a way that makes the exam fast and easy to do. There are several ways in which this can be done, depending on what's most comfortable for you. You can sit or lie down on your bed, squat or kneel on the floor, or stand up.

Most important is that you are *comfortable,* in a position that allows you to see the clearest and the most comprehensive view of your V zone in your hand-held mirror. Often this is best accomplished by sitting on your bed with your feet up and your body in a slightly reclined position, using a pillow to prop up your back.

Once you have positioned yourself, you are ready to begin. According to the Center for Vulvar Disease, here are the steps you should take:

Step 1. Viewing your vulva in the hand mirror, separate the outer lips with your fingers. A normal vulva should be pink to medium red in color, with no obvious discolorations or very light areas. You should also be on the lookout for any dark red areas, swelling (the tissue may look or feel bloated), blisters, bumps, lesions, sores, unusual colors, and particularly any unusual odors. Certainly make note of any pain you feel when touching any area of your vulva.

Step 2. Now look a little deeper inside. For this you will need to locate and then separate your *inner* lips. Look for the same signs mentioned in step 1. In addition, also check the entrance to your vagina for those signs.

Step 3. Examine your clitoris, located just under a hood or fold of skin just below the urinary opening. It should resemble a small, fleshy mound. It is soft to the touch and pink in color. Some say it resembles a tiny penis.

Step 4. Check the area outside your V zone: the urethra, perineum, anus, and the outside of the labia majora and mons veneris (see previous illustration). In addition to redness, swelling, or discolorations, check for soreness or irritation as well as itching. Certainly, pay spe-

IF THIS IS YOUR FIRST SELF-EXAM . . .

. . . experts suggest you try it directly after a gynecology visit, when your doctor has already verified your V zone health. In this way you will know that what you are looking at is normal for you. Then in future exams, you will have a point of reference—a barometer by which to gauge your findings.

cial attention to signs of bleeding (such as dried or moist blood) other than that which is associated with your monthly cycle.

Protection Plus:
How Your Doctor Can Help

If during a vulvar self-exam you discover anything that seems even a bit unusual, you should bring it to your doctor's attention, and usually the sooner, the better. In many instances, he or she will simply reassure you that everything is all right. Nevertheless, if things seem abnormal to you, ask for an explanation as well as what you should look for as a sign of trouble.

Even if your body continues to check out okay, however, it's still important that you don't skip regular gynecological exams. Indeed, while performing monthly self-exams is important, there are some instances when, despite the fact that everything looks and feels okay, something *is* terribly wrong. And that's where your doctor can play a major, sometimes life-saving, role. In fact, even when you seemingly have no problems, seeing your doctor at least once a year allows you to give yourself the gift of preventative care, and in doing so, help preserve not only your V zone health but your overall good health, as well as your sexual vitality.

Your Annual Gynecological Exam:
What It Must Include

Most experts agree that the first, most important step of any gynecological exam is the consultation—a talk between you and your doctor that should take place while you are still fully dressed. Here you should bring up any symptoms you may have discovered on your own, as well as any complaints you may have about your V zone, as well as your overall health. This is an especially important step if you see a gynecologist only once a year, for an annual exam.

This is also the time when you should ask your doctor any potentially "embarrassing" V zone questions you may have. Indeed, most women find that they feel less intimidated about asking questions when they are fully dressed, rather than undressed and in a compromising exam position. If you give it a try you may be surprised to discover how much easier it is to talk to your doctor during this preexam consult.

Once this discussion takes place and you are satisfied with the answers your doctor provides, you will proceed to the physical portion of your exam. It should include at least the following four steps:

1. The General Health Check. This should include listening to your heart and lungs and feeling your neck. You may be asked to give a urine sample, which will be tested for sugar (a sign of diabetes) or blood (a sign of infection). If your gynecologist is also your primary care doctor (and you must make a point of discussing this with your doctor, as not all feel comfortable in this total-care role), your exam should include a check of any general health concerns you mention during your consult.

2. The Breast Check. This should take up to two minutes. Your doctor should feel each breast, usually using a circular motion, examining the nipples, as well as the area under each armpit (see illustration). Since research shows that up to 25 percent of all gynecologists skip this step, it may be necessary for you to ask for this portion of the exam—and *you* must take the initiative. It's that vital to your health. In addition, if you haven't been doing self-breast exams, now is the time to 'fess up. Your doctor must know if this is the case for you.

3. The Pelvic Exam. This should begin with a check of the outside portion of your V zone. Here your doctor is looking for the same factors you look for in your vulvar self-exam: lumps, bumps, discolorations, redness, or swelling.

The next step is an internal exam. It begins with inserting the speculum, which should only cause *minimal* discomfort. If you experience pain, talk to your doctor about using a smaller instrument. Also, relaxing your pelvic muscles as much as possible will help make the exam more comfortable. Once your vagina is held open, your doctor will examine the inside of the vaginal walls and take a Pap smear. This is the screening for cervical cancer and a test that is mandatory at least every other year for all sexually active women (see

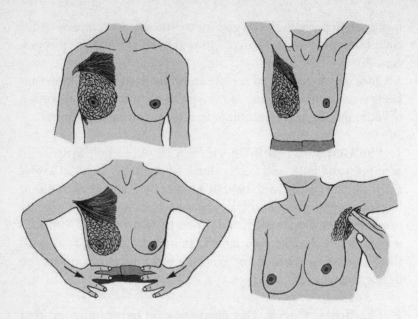

THE BREAST EXAM

A complete breast exam should be performed by your doctor at least once yearly—and more often if any abnormalities are detected. While some doctors may perform the exam while you are lying down, for a really thorough breast check you should be sitting or standing. Your doctor should check not only the breast itself, but also the surrounding muscles and tendons, including the area under both armpits. You can follow this same pattern when performing a breast self-exam.

Courtesy of Lippincott, Williams & Wilkins, Medi-Clip

"The New Pap Smear" below). This test should be followed by the bi-manual exam. Here, your doctor will place the fingers of one hand inside your vagina and the other on your stomach, and then gently feel your pelvic organs. In this way he or she can feel the shape, size, and position of your cervix, ovaries, and uterus and check for any growths such as fibroid tumors or cysts.

4. The Recto-Vaginal Exam. This is by far the most overlooked part of the exam—many doctors don't like to do it, and most women avoid it as well. Still, many experts agree it's a vital way for your doctor to check the internal area *behind* your vagina and uterus, which can often reveal problems not felt during the bimanual exam, including cysts and tumors, as well as endometriosis, tubal infections, and even polyps. For this portion of the exam, which should take less than a minute, your doctor will insert one gloved finger into your rectum. Don't be alarmed if you feel a momentary sensation of having to have a bowel movement. You won't. It's just a normal sensation.

5. The Conclusion. Every exam should conclude with a talk, where you and your doctor can discuss any problems discovered during your exam, as well as any additional tests you may need and any self-care treatments you need to do. You should also use this time to bring up any additional questions you have and discuss any treatment options. It's also a good idea to ask your doctor when you should call for test results, particularly your Pap smear. If your doctor suggests a follow-up exam for anything he or she would like to watch (such as a cyst or even an irritation), don't take the suggestion lightly, and make an appointment before you leave.

The New Pap Smear: How It Can Save Your Life

Among the most important V zone screening available today is the Pap smear. Developed in the 1940s as a way of looking for cell changes that can, if not treated, result in cervical cancer, it has been credited with saving the lives of hundreds of thousands of women throughout the years.

More recently, the Pap smear has become an even more important tool. Doctors now know that at least one sexually transmitted virus (certain strains of the human papilloma virus, or HPV—see Chapter 9) can cause cell changes that lead to cervical cancer. With the advent of the sexual revolution and the social acceptance of multiple sex partners, now, more than ever before, women have become vulnerable to contracting this virus and developing cervical cancer.

The important news is that the Pap smear is a highly effective method of discovering those who are at high risk—often early enough to save a life. And the test is getting better, with important improvements in both the way the actual screening is done and how the cells are analyzed.

Why is it important for you to know these details? In many instances, the use of the newer technologies *is not* automatic. Indeed, many of you will have to request some of these new technologies specifically before your doctor will comply. Sometimes you may even need to consider a different doctor since, unfortunately, not all physicians routinely keep up with the latest advances, including the newest ways to *save your life*. Additionally, since some doctors are coerced by managed care companies to restrict suggestions of what can be a more costly procedure, they neglect to mention all that's available to their patients.

That said, here's a rundown of the newest, most important technologies in the area of cervical screening. Remember, depending on your insurance coverage, you may have to foot the bill for the difference in cost over and above a regular Pap smear. Usually, however, this nominal expense is well worth it.

Technology: Thin Prep Test

What It Is: A new way of collecting and preparing Pap smear samples for analysis.

How It's Done: Instead of swabbing your cervix and placing the cells on a slide before sending it to the laboratory, the traditional swab or brush is replaced by a special wand that goes directly from your cervix into a vial of fluid, which is sent to the laboratory. This ensures that the entire cell sampling, and not just a small portion, is submitted for analysis. Once it reaches the lab, your sample is put through a declumping process, which makes it easier to see each of the sampled cells, and then a filtering procedure, to separate out the blood and mucus. The remaining cervical cells are then spread in a thin layer onto the glass slide for analysis. The end result is a slide that is clearer and easier to read and a diagnosis that is ultimately more accurate.

Improved Accuracy: A study of some 7,000 women conducted by the manufacturer revealed Thin Prep was able to pinpoint abnormalities 65 percent more often than the traditionally prepared Pap smear slide.

A second study on some 50,000 women published in the *Medical Journal of Australia* found Thin Prep was not only more efficient at identifying severe levels of cell abnormality, it found these abnormalities more often than the traditional Pap smear. In certain instances, Thin Prep found high-grade lesions, indicating an advanced form of cervical disease, while no such cells were seen on the traditional Pap smear, even with a second review.

Additional Cost: About $20 over and above the cost of a traditional Pap smear. Most insurance companies *won't* pick up the extra tab.

Technology: PapSure Test

What It Is: An on-site visual cervical exam performed at the same time as a traditional Pap smear.

How It's Done: Immediately after taking your Pap smear, your doctor will "wash" your cervix with a diluted solution of white table vinegar, which will adhere to abnormal cells. Then, by exposing the cervix directly to a harmless, disposable, low-glare, blue-white chemiluminescent light source (the process is called *speculoscopy*), any abnormal cells become immediately apparent to the eye. Normal cells look bluish in color; abnormal cells are distinctly white. So, your doctor can immediately tell if abnormal cells are present and where they are located.

Most often, when the PapSure test results are negative—meaning no abnormal cells are seen—the Pap smear portion of the test is negative as well, and it's a result you can comfortably believe is true. If, in rare instances, PapSure is negative but the Pap smear is positive, then your condition is considered positive until proven otherwise.

Improved Accuracy: When performed along with a traditional Pap smear, the PapSure test has been shown to be more than twice as accurate in identifying cervical abnormalities *before* they progress to cancer—a 90 percent rate for PapSure compared to a 40 percent rate with Pap smear alone. Perhaps more important, it is equally effective in ruling out cancer, meaning you can now feel highly confident about a negative Pap smear result.

Although using PapSure technology is not considered "required," the Food and Drug Administration (FDA) has allowed PapSure inventors (the Trylon Corporation) to say that the exam is *indicated* in all women undergoing a pelvic exam and Pap smear—meaning that there is enough evidence to show it's worth the extra effort. Another bonus for you is that PapSure offers an immediate diagnosis, meaning there's no waiting for test results.

Additional Cost: About $25 over and above the cost of your regular Pap. Most insurance companies do not pay.

Technology: AutoPap and PAPNET
What It Is: Automated methods of analyzing Pap smear slides.

How It's Done: In both tests computers are used to read the Pap smear slides, helping to decrease the margin of human error. In PAPNET the slides are reread by the computer after first being seen by a cytologist. In AutoPap, the slides are read by computer analysis first, and those that indicate an abnormality are reread by a cytologist.

Improved Accuracy of PAPNET: Studies comparing positive PAPNET test results with those obtained by the traditional manual screening method were similar in number. The PAPNET, however, was faster. Additionally, studies conducted in 1997 on some 21,000 women and reported in the journal *Lancet* found that PAPNET was able to identify negative smears 77 percent of the time versus 42 percent using traditional manual reading techniques. A 1998 American study published in the journal *Obstetrics and Gynecology* found PAPNET useful as a second analysis when Pap smears were classified as containing atypical squamous cells of undetermined origin (often identified on test results as "ASCUS"). Specifically, PAPNET was able to determine which women needed treatment to obliterate their abnormal cells and which were likely to experience a regression back to normal cell status on their own—all without a biopsy.

AN EXPERT'S OPINION ON . . .

Avoiding Pap Smear Mistakes

While most women believe the greatest number of Pap smear errors are due to incorrect interpretation of the slides, according to Dr. William Rich, clinical professor of obstetrics and gynecology at the University of California, San Francisco, the major error really lies in mistakenly believing the Pap smear *screening* is really a *diagnostic test*. What's the difference between the two? According to Dr. Rich, a negative *diagnostic test* can rule out a problem such as cancer; a negative *screening* cannot. In terms of a Pap smear, Rich says that sometimes there can be so much uterine inflammation that the only samples that make it on to the Pap smear slide are cellular debris. This, in turn, can keep the pathologist from seeing the cancer cells. He says "When a woman has symptoms such as bleeding after intercourse, bleeding between periods, or a foul, watery discharge, then cancer of the cervix must be excluded. [And] only a thorough examination and biopsy can rule out a cervical cancer." He adds that if you have these symptoms, "Never, never, never, ever accept a normal Pap test as proof of there being no cancer."

Also remember that an abnormal Pap smear is *not* a diagnosis, so it should *never* lead directly to treatment. Instead, says Rich, all abnormal Pap smears must be followed by a diagnostic measure such as a biopsy or colposcopy (an internal examination using a specially designed microscope). Never, he says, accept a hysterectomy based on an abnormal Pap smear reading alone.

Improved Accuracy of AutoPap: Data from a large-scale clinical study of Pap smears taken from more than 25,000 patients from five different laboratories found that AutoPap achieved greater accuracy in early diagnosis of cervical disease and reduced incidence of both false-positive and false-negative results.

Added Cost: Both PAPNET and AutoPap add about $35 each to the cost of a Pap smear. Most insurance plans don't cover it.

How You Can Make Every Pap Test Count

Regardless of what your doctor may do to help increase the accuracy of your Pap smear, there are steps you can take as well to ensure a more accurate test result. According to the American Society of Clinical Pathologists (ASCP)—the folks that read your Pap smear tests—and experts from the Virginia Mason Medical Center in Seattle, here's what to do:

- Schedule your gynecologic exam at the optimum time, usually two weeks after the first day of your last menstrual cycle. Estrogen levels are highest at this time, making the cell samples easier to read and interpret. Never have a Pap smear during a menstrual period.
- Don't put anything in your vagina for at least twenty-four hours (ASCP suggests seventy-two hours) prior to your Pap smear. This includes vaginal medications, creams, contraceptive foams or jellies including spermicide, douches, and tampons. You should also abstain from intercourse for twenty-four hours prior to your test.
- Never have a Pap smear when you are experiencing signs of a vaginal infection, such as unusual discharge or itching. A yeast infection can be particularly disruptive since it often causes an increase in inflammation and cell changes that make the test difficult to read.
- Ask your doctor where he or she is sending your sample for analysis—and make certain the laboratory is accredited, employing nationally certified cytotechnologists and board certified pathologists.
- Have a Pap smear every year, beginning as soon as you are sexually active, or at least by age eighteen. Despite common misconcep-

tions, all women, including lesbians and those who are not in-volved in any kind of sexual relationship, need an annual Pap smear.

ON THE HORIZON: THE TEST THAT MAY REPLACE THE PAP SMEAR

If a group of British researchers are right, we may have a brand-new way to test for cervical cancer—one that could eliminate Pap smear test errors by a significant margin. Called the Campaign Test (in honor of the Cancer Research Campaign at Cambridge University, where the test was developed), it uses a fluorescent dye to highlight antibodies designed to home in on abnormal cells on a cervical smear. The fluorescent marker is then able to separate ir-regular from regular cells, and make them clearly visible. Accord-ing to a BBC News report, preliminary results indicate the new test is 100 percent efficient at detecting abnormal cervical cells. If further studies prove the test is more effective than the Pap smear, it could be available in the United States within five years.

The HPV Test and Cervical Cancer

Many doctors believe that the most accurate way of detecting cervical cancer is to test for something else entirely: HPV, the human papil-loma virus. The reason? Studies now show that certain strains of the virus are present in virtually 100 percent of all cases of cervical cancer. While the latest study—a January 2000 report in the *Journal of the American Medical Association*—reveals that testing for HPV has a higher false-positive rate than the traditional Pap smear, many believe that in time the test will be refined enough to become the gold stan-dard for cervical cancer, particularly in women over age thirty-five. One factor that certainly makes the HPV test attractive is that it in-volves only a simple swabbing of the vagina, which a woman can eas-ily do on her own. The tissue is then analyzed for DNA from thirteen different types of suspect strains of HPV. (For more information on HPV, cervical cancer, and this test, see Chapter 8.)

Becoming a Savvy Medical Consumer: What You Must Do Now

Now that you know a little something about how your V zone functions, you will be well prepared to understand and act on the information that is found in the remainder of this book, much of which you will need to maintain optimum intimate health. In many instances, I hope you will also find answers to your intimate care questions—subjects that for a variety of reasons you may have found difficult to discuss with your own doctor. Indeed, whether it is simple shyness on your part that's kept you in the dark or, as is more often the case, your doctor is simply not as approachable about intimate care subjects as you would hope he or she would be, if you're not getting the answers you need, your health care can suffer.

Just having all this information, however, isn't quite enough. You must put it to use by becoming the single most proactive element in your health care. Indeed, if you are to obtain and maintain the best V zone care, *you* must become involved—not only in selecting the doctor who will care for you but also in deciding on the types of treatments you will receive throughout the course of that care. The information you find in this book can help you achieve that. By sharing what you learn with your own gynecologist, you can open a dialogue about your V zone health that will be of value not only today but also far into your future.

The bottom line is this: Only when you and your doctor work together as a team will you be assured of getting the best care possible. And this V zone guide *will* help you become the *best team player possible*!

CHAPTER TWO

Coping with BV

The Latest News on Bacterial Vaginosis

Chances are that you've already experienced at least one episode of the burning, itching, V zone irritation known as vaginitis, the single most common health problem affecting women today. One reason it is such a frequent diagnosis is that *vaginitis* is a broad term used to describe a variety of vaginal conditions. Indeed, everything from simple irritations caused by bath products or lubricants all the way up to complex infections that can seriously jeopardize your health have been called vaginitis.

However, according to the National Vaginitis Association (NVA), for many women in their reproductive years, a diagnosis of vaginitis commonly means an infection known as bacterial vaginosis, or BV. Although a potentially serious infection caused by any number of different bacteria, when treated early on, usually with a simple regimen of highly effective medications, it is easily cured with few, if any, lingering complications.

When, however, left undiagnosed or untreated for even a short time, BV can not only dramatically increase your risk of pelvic inflammatory disease, or PID, a potentially life-threatening infection that can also destroy your fertility (see Chapter 7), it can also increase your risk of contracting numerous sexually transmitted diseases, including HIV, the virus that causes AIDS.

The latest research also shows that BV may, in fact, also have links to cervical cancer, thus increasing risks there as well. Finally, should you contract BV during pregnancy, a whole list of complications is possible, some that can seriously jeopardize your baby's life.

If you've never heard of BV, you're not alone. Surveys show that many women are unfamiliar with the term. One reason is that until fairly recently, BV was known as "nonspecific vaginitis" or sometimes "gardnerella," after one of the bacteria often associated with this infection. The name was changed to BV only after researchers began to see how many different bacteria were capable of triggering the same vaginal symptoms and ultimately leading to similar complications.

How BV Develops

One of the ways in which your vagina stays healthy and disease free is by a natural feminine ecosystem that is ingeniously designed to foster good health. What makes it all work is a complex balance of many micro-organisms (some of which can cause vaginitis) that work together in a unique system of checks and balances to make sure no one specific factor can begin growing out of control.

The so-called gatekeeper of the whole system is a "good" bacteria known as *lactobacillus*. By breaking down certain chemicals in the vagina, it helps your body maintain a highly acidic V zone environment. Since most nasty, disease-causing bacteria hate acid, this environment helps ensure that your vagina remains healthy. Increasing the effectiveness even more is the fact that some forms of lactobacillus also emit a powerful germ-fighting chemical known as hydrogen peroxide, which also helps keep your vagina healthy, particularly if any bacteria are introduced into your body.

The newest study in this area, joint research between doctors in Kenya, Africa, and the University of Washington in Seattle, reported in the December 1999 *Journal of Infectious Diseases,* found that the presence of lactobacillus in the vagina, in the proper amount, may actually reduce the risk of infection from a number of STDs, including gonorrhea and even HIV.

Unfortunately, however, the power of lactobacillus can be overturned and the amounts needed for optimal health may not always be available. Although any number of circumstances can contribute to this—stress, allergies, hormones, medication, even a change in diet—when it comes to BV, many researchers believe that our sex life may play a unique but important role.

Sex, BV, and the Vagina Virus: The Newest Links

Because BV overwhelmingly occurs in women who are sexually active, many doctors long suspected that sex is the real culprit behind this infection. Adding fuel to that fire, a nationwide study of women being treated for STDs at clinics around the nation revealed that up to 64 percent were also diagnosed with BV. Studies elsewhere showed that women who already had BV appeared to be at greater risk for contracting an STD, particularly gonorrhea and chlamydia. More recently, research on some 200 women conducted at Johns Hopkins School of Public Health revealed that women with BV were nearly four times more likely to contract HIV.

Although all this information was clearly indicating links between sexual activity and BV, there remained one nagging question: Which came first: the sex or the infection? Moreover, doctors became increasingly interested in whether BV could result from sex with even a seemingly healthy partner.

At least part of this question was answered in early 1999 when an international team of experts, headed by a prominent *female scientist,* discovered the first evidence that a sexually transmitted *"vagina virus"* may in fact be the real cause of BV. Remarkably, it was an organism with just one purpose: to destroy the "good" lactobacillus bacteria that keep the vagina healthy.

The study, which included some 200 women from three major medical centers (the University of Chicago, Baylor College of Medicine in Texas, and the University of Trabzon in Turkey), used DNA fingerprinting and other sophisticated technologies to isolate the virus in various strains of infected lactobacillus. Although the bacterial strains themselves were slightly different for each of the women, the infecting virus appeared to be the same in almost all of them.

So how did these women get the virus in the first place? If you're guessing that their partners were a potential source, you're right. An analysis of male urine samples reviewed during the study found at least two strains of lactobacillus that were capable of killing at least eleven strains of the protective lactobacillus women need to maintain vaginal health. Whether all men carry these strains naturally or they are the result of some other infection or problem in their body, no one could say.

Still, the evidence linking sex and BV was now finally strong enough to forge a true *scientific* connection. Specifically, the new "vagina virus" transmitted during intimate contact appeared to be at least one of the more important factors involved in BV.

Although this research represented a giant leap forward in understanding how and why BV occurs, it didn't tell the whole story. The reason is that although most women who get this infection are sexually active, this is not a hard-and-fast rule. Some were clearly active in the past, leading researchers to theorize that the vagina virus could lie dormant in some women for a number of years, but some who developed BV had no sexual experiences at all.

Doctors suspected that there had to be yet another compounding factor that was allowing the vagina virus to get into the body or, more likely, that some other factor altogether was responsible for some cases of BV. For many, that factor was beginning to look like the common feminine hygiene practice of douching.

Indeed, a recent study published in the *Journal of Infectious Diseases* found that douching can increase the risk of BV by some 50 percent, making those women who douche regularly twice as likely to get this infection. No one is certain how or why, but researchers theorize that the douching process alters the vaginal environment and disrupts the natural ecosystem, causing the "good" lactobacillus to plummet and allowing any "bad" bacteria present in the vagina to take hold. Additionally, studies show that if any mild infections are present in the vagina at the time of douching, they can be driven deeper into the reproductive system, thus increasing the risk of not only BV but other complications, including PID.

Could You Have BV? How to Tell

Although you may never know exactly why your BV infection has occurred, the more quickly you are diagnosed and treated, the lower your risk is of developing any serious complications. The best way to ensure that this is the case is to pay close attention to symptoms that signal a problem. According to the NVA, look for the following signs:

Vaginal discharge—Usually thin, watery, milky-white or gray in color, it may also have a somewhat sticky feel. You may also notice the amount of discharge is significantly more than in the past.

Vaginal odor—Often described as foul smelling, or fishy.

Offensive odors or discharge that grow worse after intercourse.

Occasional itching or burning but with little signs of inflammation.

You might think that these symptoms are so obvious that spotting BV is easy, but it's easy to be fooled. In some women symptoms can be so subtle they can easily go unnoticed, particularly at the start of an infection. Indeed, studies show that up to 50 percent of women diagnosed with BV by their doctor never noticed any symptoms.

At the same time, if you are relying solely on your doctor to diagnose your BV, there are a few things you should know. First, neither a routine pelvic exam nor even a Pap smear can necessarily spot BV. Indeed, specific tests are necessary in order for a truly accurate diagnosis. Moreover, even if your doctor suspects BV symptoms during an exam (such as discharge or odor), studies show he or she *might not* offer testing or treatment. According to a recent NVA survey, unless a patient brings BV symptoms to her doctor's attention, many physicians simply overlook even blatant signs of this infection observable during the exam. Why is this so?

One reason is that in the past, doctors believed BV infections were so harmless that it almost didn't matter whether they were treated.

Today we know how wrong this kind of thinking is. Unfortunately, not all doctors are equally versed on the latest research.

Indeed, the complications of not only BV but all other vaginal infections are now considered so important that the American College of Obstetricians and Gynecologists (ACOG) recently issued a stern warning to its members to begin taking a more aggressive stance in diagnosing and treating these diseases. They urged women to be more vigilant in this area as well. "Women should not underestimate their risk for common infections that have serious complications," noted Ralph W. Hale, M.D., executive vice president of ACOG.

The BV Tests: What You Might Need

Identifying all forms of vaginitis requires at least two tests: one that reads the pH, or the acid level, of your vagina and one that analyzes fresh samples of discharge for specific bacteria. In some instances your doctor may send the specimens to a laboratory for analysis; in other instances part or all of the analysis may be performed immediately in the doctor's office. In either case, here's what to expect.

To test pH, your doctor will swab the inside of your vagina and place the fluid onto color-treated litmus paper. The color that the paper changes to after the fluids are added helps determine the acid or pH level. Normal pH can range from 4.5 to 5.5. When it rises higher than 5.5, acid levels are said to be low, a condition that favors BV. When pH falls below 4.5, acid levels are high, a condition that generally discourages BV—but can increase the risk of other types of problems. You are optimally looking for that normal pH range to show that everything is all right.

Next, your doctor will swab samples of your vaginal discharge and place them on two separate microscopic slides. On one slide, your fluids are diluted with a saline (saltwater) solution; the second slide contains a potassium mixture. If the slide containing the potassium gives off an odor (called the "whiff" test), either BV or a second infection, called trichomoniasis (see Chapter 7), is usually present.

If either the pH or the whiff test is positive, the slides must then be examined under a microscope to verify BV. In BV, a specific amount

---

BV TEST WARNING

A disturbing new survey of more than 300 gynecologists revealed that the majority do not use the most efficient testing methods for BV: the combined pH, whiff tests, and slide analysis. Only 42 percent of the doctors reported testing pH, and 15 percent admitted they frequently "diagnosed BV" by telephone only. Moreover, 43 percent said they used Pap smears to diagnose BV, and 28 percent relied on cultures of vaginal fluids, although neither of these tests is considered reliable for diagnosing bacterial vaginosis.

For that reason, you should be extra vigilant about making certain your doctor performs *all* necessary testing—and don't accept a telephone diagnosis. In addition, ask your doctor what specific tests he or she is taking, and get specific results. If you're not satisfied with the answers—and especially if your symptoms linger on—seek at least one more medical opinion.

---

of "clue" cells (cells from the lining of the vagina with a particular look) will appear on the slide containing the saline. If they don't, your symptoms could be the result of a yeast infection (see Chapter 3), or, if no bacteria are present, caused by an irritation from factors outside your body—such as panty hose, or some intimate care products (see Chapter 9).

The FemExam: The Newest Way to Test for BV

A brand-new test specifically developed for vaginal infections may mean not only a faster but an easier and more accurate diagnosis. Called the FemExam, it uses a chemically prepared test card (about the size of credit card) onto which your doctor drops tiny samples of vaginal fluid. Chemicals embedded in the card measure not only your vaginal pH level but also the chemicals responsible for the odors detected on the whiff test—a method that is thought to be far more reliable than just smell alone. To help make diagnosis even easier, instead of relying on just color changes to indicate the important reactions, the FemExam uses plus and minus signs appearing in different colors.

In addition, a second FemExam has been developed specifically for BV. It measures vaginal fluids for levels of an enzyme known as PIP (proline iminopeptidase), which increases in response to BV. What makes the FemExam particularly helpful is that it has a built-in sys-

AN EXPERT'S OPINION ON . . .

Pap Smears and BV: An Important Connection

While a Pap smear won't diagnose a BV infection, there could be an important connection. According to experts at a roundtable discussion at the Interscience Conference on Antimicrobial Agents and Chemotherapy, BV may affect a Pap smear in a variety of ways. Specifically, a BV infection may cause a false-positive Pap smear reading. This can occur when clue cells from the BV infection make it more difficult to read the status of the cervical cells used for the Pap smear accurately. Indeed, several studies have shown an increase in inflammatory Pap smears in women with BV. Since most of the time, a Pap smear that indicates inflammation or the presence of atypical cells must be repeated within three to six months, many experts now suggest that testing, and particularly treatment for BV, should take place in the interim—even if there are no obvious symptoms present at the time.

If you receive an abnormal Pap smear reading, and particularly if you are also experiencing some symptoms of BV, be certain to talk to your doctor about further testing and treatment before your next Pap smear.

tem of checks and balances that not only verify test results but also that the card itself is activated and working.

In comparison tests, the FemExam was found to produce results equal to or better than the traditional testing methods. This may mean not only a more accurate test (one that leaves less open for interpretation) but also an immediate answer about your symptoms— as well as the opportunity to begin treatment right away.

Although many doctors already incorporate the FemExam into their regular diagnostic and treatment regimen, not all do. Thus, feel free to bring this test option to your doctor's attention and ask for his or her thoughts as to whether it can help you. Since most insurance companies don't cover the extra cost (it will likely be built in to your doctor's fee), some doctors won't perform the extra step unless a patient requests it. Certainly if it's already in your doctor's treatment arsenal, you should have the option of having the test.

When BV Is Diagnosed: The Treatments That Can Help

The goal of all BV treatments is to reduce levels of the nasty bacteria causing the infection without harming levels of the "good" lactobacillus bacteria. According to a report issued by the American Academy of Family Physicians, the following medications have been shown to do just that.

Oral metronidazole. The most common prescription for BV, it is often administered in 500 mg pills, taken two times a day for seven days. An alternate version is a single 2-gram dose. Although this option is easier—you don't have to remember to take any pills—any sensitivity or side effects may be magnified because the dosage is so high. Do note, however, that the medicine used in the one-dose treatment is formulated differently from the multidose treatment, and you cannot get the desired effect by simply taking your entire seven-day prescription in one day. In fact doing so could be dangerous. If you want the one-dose treatment, tell your doctor and get a prescription specifically for that drug. Do note, however, that clinical studies show the cure rate for the seven-day regimen is 95 percent, while the rate of recovery using the one-dose method drops to 84 percent.

Potential side effects: The most serious side effects are seizures and numbness, particularly in the arms, legs, hands, and feet. More common effects are stomach cramps, constipation, diarrhea, headache, nausea, and vomiting.

Metronidazole cream (2% strength). A 5-gram application (in a premeasured applicator) once a day at bedtime for seven days.

Potential side effects: Same as for oral metronidazole.

Metronidazole gel (.75% strength). Applied intravaginally twice a day for five days.

Potential side effects: Stomach cramps, uterine cramping, inflammation of the cervix or vagina, genital itching, metallic or "bad taste" in the mouth, nausea.

Clindamycin cream (2%). One full applicator (5 grams) intravaginally, once a day at bedtime, for seven days. A newer version of this drug now requires only a three-day treatment regimen. It is not approved for use in pregnancy. The seven-day version can be used by both pregnant and nonpregnant women. In addition, clinical trials have shown that an oral version of clindamycin—300 mg two times a day for seven days—is also effective, although widespread experience is still somewhat limited.

Potential side effects: Inflammation of the cervix, vagina, vulva, frothy or yellow discharge with burning and itching. Ironically, treatment with clindamycin may increase the risk of yeast infection.

BV DRUGS: SPECIAL WARNINGS

While taking medication for a BV infection, be certain to avoid alcohol. In addition, try to avoid intercourse, or if you do have relations, use a condom. Do not use tampons while using topical medications for BV, since they can absorb much of the drug and decrease effectiveness.

AN EXPERT'S OPINION ON . . .

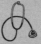

BV and Your Partner

Q: My BV infections keep recurring. Would it help if my partner received treatment at the same time?

A: Unfortunately, no. According to the Sexually Transmitted Disease Information Center provided by the *Journal of the American Medical Association,* treatment of the male partner does not appear to be beneficial in preventing a woman's recurrence of BV or in hastening her recovery—mainly because infections do not appear to exist in a man's body. However, in light of the new information concerning the role of the vagina virus in the development of BV, which can come from your partner, you might want to consider using a condom for several months, to reduce the risk of transmission. This may help reduce your risk of recurring BV infection.

BV and Pregnancy

While obstetricians have long suspected that BV may in fact be linked to problems in pregnancy, in 1995 a large-scale study of more than 10,000 women from seven medical centers in five different United States cities proved their fears were not unfounded.

The research, jointly funded by the National Institute of Child Health and Human Development (NICHD) and the National Institute of Allergy and Infectious Diseases (NIAID), and published in the *New England Journal of Medicine,* found that pregnant women who were diagnosed with BV during their second trimester were up to 40 percent more likely to deliver a premature baby, with significantly low birth weight—under five pounds. Other variables that could affect the study outcome, such as smoking, race, and previous delivery of a preterm baby, were taken into consideration, and still BV was found to be a significant contributing factor.

This study echoes findings of a 1993 report in the *American Journal of Obstetrics and Gynecology,* noting that women with BV had a higher incidence of premature rupture of the pregnancy membrane, leading to early delivery.

Although researchers aren't certain why BV is linked to preterm birth, many believe that in addition to causing a vaginal infection, the offending bacteria may invade the uterus, triggering the premature labor.

Additionally, NICHD studies published in 1996 in the *Journal of Obstetrics and Gynecology* found BV was also linked to higher-than-normal levels of fetal fibronectin, a biochemical that's produced naturally during pregnancy and in excessive amounts can lead to premature labor.

If you are pregnant, experts say you must bring any threat of BV symptoms to the attention of your obstetrician immediately. Don't wait for him or her to make the diagnosis on their own.

According to one researcher who worked on the study, Sharon Hillier, Ph.D., "this very common vaginal syndrome is not routinely diagnosed in pregnant women currently because many physicians have not really appreciated that this very common vaginal complaint could be a cause of complications in pregnancy." Indeed, since research linking BV and pregnancy outcome is still considered new, many physicians are unaware that the link exists.

However, says Hillier, the data from the new studies is so sound that all women with symptoms should definitely be screened for these infections during pregnancy. Some experts believe the links are so strong that it warrants testing all pregnant women, even when no symptoms exist.

Miscarriage and BV

Among the newest concerns about BV is that it may increase the risk of miscarriage, particularly in the early stages of pregnancy. According to Dr. Susan Ralph and colleagues from Leeds General Infirmary in London, England, while BV does not appear to affect getting pregnant, it was linked to a twofold increase in the risk of pregnancy loss during the first trimester. Reporting in the *British Medical Journal,* the doctors say that in their study of over 850 women, 31.6 percent with BV had an increased risk of miscarriage, as compared to just a little over 18 percent who did not harbor the infection. While the experts are not clear exactly how or why BV encourages miscarriage, they suggest it may be due to an inflammation inside the uterus that exists at the time of implantation, thus making it difficult for the baby to attach to the mother's body, and ultimately, to survive.

Treating BV During Pregnancy: Special Precautions

Because BV can significantly affect the outcome of pregnancy, infections that occur during this time must be treated. However, according to the Centers for Disease Control (CDC), because metronidazole has been shown in laboratory studies to increase the risk of birth defects, particularly during the first three months of pregnancy, you should avoid this medication, particularly during your first trimester.

In addition, because residues of metronidazole have been found in breast milk, you should avoid this drug while you are breast-feeding. If treatment is necessary, stop breast-feeding while you are taking this medication. Because studies on pregnancy and the gel and cream versions of metronidazole are still considered inconclusive, many experts advise that you also avoid these medications during pregnancy—or if you are actively trying to conceive.

Although no studies have shown clindamycin to cause birth defects, studies are also considered inconclusive. If you are pregnant or planning to conceive, make certain your gynecologist knows before prescribing any medication for BV.

When Your BV Just Won't Quit: What to Do

For many women, a single BV infection is all they will ever experience in their lifetime. For others, however, BV may recur over and

AN EXPERT'S OPINION ON . . .

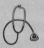

Cancer and BV: What You Must Know

New disclosures about the risks of BV are giving women still another cause for concern. Specifically, a group of researchers from Sahlgrenska University Hospital in Sweden identified a disturbing link between this vaginal infection and cervical cancer. The study, involving some 6,000 women, found BV in 10 percent, or nearly 600 patients, 5 percent of whom were also found to be harboring cervical cancer. Among the women who tested negative for BV, only a scant 1.4 percent were diagnosed with cancer. Even more disturbing, among the women with BV, another 3 percent were found to have late-stage cancer. In the BV-free group, less than ½ percent were affected with late-stage disease.

The cancer-BV link was found, say experts, thanks to something called the triple Pap smear, widely used in Scandinavian countries. Here, Pap smear samples are swabbed not just from the cervix but also the vagina.

Although no one is certain why the correlation between the two diseases exists, a recent panel of experts at the Interscience Conference of Antimicrobial Agents and Chemotherapy speculated on the possibility that BV may alter the cervix in such a way as to increase a woman's risk of HPV, the virus already linked to cervical cancer.

over, sometimes for months or even years on end. Because no one knows for certain all the factors that increase the risk of this disease, it's difficult to create a prevention strategy.

One way to guard against a recurrence is to make certain your current infection is totally cleared—and the best way to do that is by taking your complete prescription, even if symptoms disappear sooner than expected. Additionally, if symptoms are better but not gone by the time your prescription is finished, don't renew it without talking to your doctor first. It's possible your BV may have been misdiagnosed, or you developed a secondary or even a different infection. There is also a possibility that stubborn symptoms, particularly itching, may be the result of the medication rather than a lingering infection.

Discussing all these factors with your doctor will help to ensure that whatever infection you do have is totally cured, even if you need a different or a more potent medication.

A Final Word . . . Plus Ten Ways to Decrease Your Risk of BV

Even with expert medical care, sometimes BV can occur or even recur. Your best defense is to remain critically aware of your own body, particularly the symptoms of BV—and report them to your doctor right away. If he or she does not respond with testing and care, then seek a second opinion. The complications associated with untreated BV can take an enormous toll on your health, as well as severely compromising your ability to get pregnant in the future.

In addition, you should never try to treat BV on your own, even if you think you know what is wrong. Why? First, over-the-counter products won't work, so you will always need a doctor's prescription in order to cure your infection. Moreover, making the wrong diagnosis could have disastrous results, particularly when it involves self-medication. Indeed, one study showed that using a yeast treatment in the presence of BV causes a proliferation of bacteria that will literally take over your vagina in less than twenty-four hours, making any infection that existed before that much more virulent.

If you're thinking that the signs of BV are so obvious it's highly unlikely you'll confuse it with something else, guess again. According to a survey of 390 gynecologists conducted by the Institute for Epidemiological Research, nearly half of patients diagnosed with BV by their doctor had previously diagnosed themselves as having a yeast infection, and they were obviously wrong. In a subsequent study of 111 American women, 67 percent who thought they had a yeast infection in reality did not.

That said, you should also be aware that there are some things you can do on your own to help *reduce* the risk of a BV infection or help any that does exist clear somewhat faster. According to a number of medical experts, here are some things you can try:

- Wear cotton underwear. By absorbing perspiration, cotton undies can help keep your vaginal area dry, and that may help reduce the rate at which bacteria multiply.
- Change underwear frequently—at least once daily, or more frequently if it becomes soiled.
- Wear panty hose with a cotton crotch—and avoid them altogether when you can.
- Wear loose-fitting pants and shorts. Remove exercise clothes as quickly as you can after finishing your workout.
- Wash your vulva every day using unscented soap, and dry completely before getting dressed.
- Don't douche—even with water.
- After bowel movements, wipe from front to back, not back to front.
- Avoid genital sprays, deodorants, and perfumes.
- Don't sit in a wet bathing suit for long periods of time.
- Change feminine pads frequently; avoid tampons if you have an active infection.

CHAPTER THREE
The V Fungus
The Yeast of Your Worries

It itches; it burns; it can even hurt. And sometimes it won't go away, no matter what you do.

The problem is a vaginal yeast infection—another form of vaginitis that affects millions of women each year. Indeed, the latest studies show that up to 75 percent of *all* women experience at least one yeast infection during their lifetime, and nearly half of us will get it twice or more. For some, infections are on "instant replay"—one occurring right after the next, making vaginal health seem like a distant memory.

And if you think you're hearing more about the "yeastie beasties" than ever before, you're probably right. Statistics show that between 1980 and 1990, the rate of infection more than doubled, mostly due to an increase in the associated risk factors, including the use of antibiotics, birth control pills, and sexual activity (all of which you'll learn more about shortly). Of most concern is that the increase in the number of women getting yeast infections appears to be continuing.

While in itself a yeast infection is not life threatening, it can certainly be uncomfortable. Moreover, when left untreated for an extended period of time, it can increase your risk of other V zone infections, including some sexually transmitted diseases—infections that can ultimately destroy your fertility.

Because of that, it's a good idea to learn not only about how and why yeast infections occur but, more important, what you can do to reduce your risks and, when necessary, eliminate symptoms as fast as possible.

Do You Have a Yeast Infection? How to Tell

As you read earlier, the health of your entire V zone is affected by a highly precise feminine ecosystem. In order to remain disease free, it must maintain a delicate balance of a variety of micro-organisms including several species of a fungus called candidiasis—what we commonly know as yeast. Normally present in small amounts in all women, it is the "good" lactobacillus bacteria that help keep the fungus from growing out of control.

When, however, something causes lactobacillus levels to fall or in some other way alters the vaginal environment (and you'll find out *what* causes this as you read on), the candidiasis fungus can begin to multiply. Often it is only a matter of days until symptoms appear and a yeast infection is in full swing.

According to the Centers for Disease Control's STD Information Center, for most women the classic and often the most obvious sign of a yeast infection is a distinct white, clumpy discharge—what doctors often describe as resembling cottage cheese. Generally odor free (although some women insist they detect the smell of freshly baked bread!), it can also take on a yellow or tan color if a second V zone infection is occurring at the same time.

Oddly enough, however, for some women a yeast discharge so closely resembles natural vaginal secretions that it is often overlooked as a symptom. To help make the distinction, there are other V zone signs that can help clue you in that something is wrong:

- Itching that is often intense and worsens the longer the infection remains untreated.
- Redness, with the inside lips of your vagina turning a bright red or purple-red.
- Soreness in and around the vagina. Sometimes related to scratching (when it breaks open the surface of delicate V zone skin), sore-

YEAST INFECTION—
OR OVERLY SENSITIVE
VAGINA? HOW TO TELL

While your symptoms may scream "yeast infection," experts warn not to jump to diagnostic conclusions. The reason? In some women, similar problems (including redness, itching, and even discharge) are really the result of extra-sensitive skin on the inside and outside of the V zone. When vaginal tissue comes in contact with acids, particularly those found in urine, the irritating symptoms flare.

If you suspect this may be your problem, particularly if you are not experiencing the characteristic clumpy white discharge, experts suggest coating your vulva with a thin layer of Vaseline once or twice a day to help protect vaginal tissue from the acid secretions. If the treatment helps, then it's likely your problem is one of sensitivity. If it doesn't, and particularly if symptoms temporarily worsen, then an infection is likely in the works.

Do remember, however, that Vaseline destroys latex, so be certain not to apply this treatment in conjunction with condom use.

ness also occurs when the infection causes tiny fissures, or cracks, in the tissue inside the vagina.

- Vulvar burn or burning on urination, which develops when tiny cracks in the tissue become inflamed from the acid content of urine.
- Painful intercourse, usually as a result of the inflamed tissue.

Six Super-Yeast Triggers—
and How to Control Them

While the exact cause of *your* personal yeast infection may be different from that of your sister or your best friend, many women do have certain trigger factors in common—conditions or situations that are known to upset the feminine ecosystem and make it easier for yeast to thrive. The good news is that for each of these risk factors, there are also countermeasures you can take—actions that can reduce the chance of subsequent infections occurring.

Here's what to look out for—and the countermeasures you can take.

Risk #1—Antibiotics: Among the most frequent causes of yeast infections are the medications you take to cure other health problems, such as a sore throat or a respiratory infection. The problem here is that the drugs do too good a job of killing bacteria—meaning that along with the "bad" bacteria making you sick, they can also kill the "good" lactobacillus bacteria you need to protect against a yeast infection. The result is that you may shake that sore throat, but you can end up with a vaginal yeast infection—one that is not likely to clear, even with treatment, until *after* your antibiotic regimen is completed.

Countermeasure: If you have suffered from an antibiotic-related yeast infection in the past, talk to your doctor about preventative care. Specifically, in the event that you need antibiotics again, find out which yeast treatments are safe and effective to use at the same time. Do not, however, combine any yeast medication, particularly oral drugs, with an antibiotic without your doctor's okay. Some work together; others do not. In addition, you might want to explore the natural route to prevention, including eating yogurt containing live acidophilus bacteria (which help increase the amount of the good lactobacillus bacteria) as well as applying it locally in your vagina. You'll learn more about the powers of yogurt over yeast infections later in this chapter.

Risk #2—Douching: While douching won't kill the good lactobacillus, it can wash it away. This changes the local environment directly in the vagina, which then makes it easier for the yeast to begin growing.

Countermeasure: Don't douche. Although some alternative medicine proponents frequently suggest a highly acidic douche (like vinegar and water), most gynecologists say douching strictly for the sake of hygiene should be avoided, particularly if you have had yeast infections in the past.

Risk #3—Birth control pills: Not only can oral contraceptives decrease the amount of acid in your vagina (causing the pH level to rise and lactobacillus level to drop), according to Dr. Thomas Shin, assistant clinical professor of obstetrics and gynecology at New York-Presbyterian Hospital, the high hormone levels found in some pills can contribute to the growth of yeast as well.

Countermeasure: If your first infection develops *after* beginning the Pill and infections continue to recur, talk to your doctor about changing your contraceptive prescription—perhaps to a lower-dose pill or even to a different type. If all else fails, experts say consider other forms of birth control.

Risk #4—IUD (intrauterine birth control device): The main problem here, says Dr. Shin, is that any foreign body residing in your body for an extended period of time can easily upset your V zone ecosystem, particularly the acid level. This increases your risk of a yeast infection. In some women, this can happen within weeks or even days of inserting an IUD; for others, problems may not appear for months or even years afterward.

Countermeasure: Certainly if you develop your first yeast infection soon after receiving your IUD, see your doctor immediately for treatment. If the infection clears and doesn't recur, then it's probably okay to leave your IUD in place. If infections continually return, back to the doctor you go—this time to discuss an alternate form of birth control, such as a diaphragm. Although this too is a foreign body, it is not a permanent implant, so the risk of upsetting your ecosystem is far less. Additionally, if your recurring yeast infections begin years after receiving your IUD, still consider it a possible source, particularly if no other reason for your infections can be found.

Risk #5—Spermicides, contraceptive foams, jellies, sex enhancement products: In addition to creating a localized allergic reaction that can eventually lead to an infection, some of these products can also have a direct effect on your ecosystem, decreasing acid levels and making it easier for yeast to grow. Additionally, certain taste-related items used for sexual enhancement, such as whipped cream or flavored lubricants, can deposit so much sugar in your vagina that if left for a period of time, they may encourage yeast to multiply—not to mention some dangerous bacteria, as well.

Countermeasure: Eliminate the use of all vaginal products for at least two weeks. Then begin testing each one individually for several

AN EXPERT'S OPINION ON . . .

Tight Jeans, Scanty Panties, and Yeast

Can what you wear increase your risk of a yeast infection—or cause one you already have to recur? Doctors say yes. Indeed, according to experts from the Yeast Infection Resource Center, any clothing that is particularly tight will cause the vagina to sweat and decrease the flow of air in the genital region—and that causes the warm, moist environment that yeast loves.

Dr. D. Ashley Hill, associate director of Obstetrics and Gynecology at Florida Hospital Family Practice Residency, warns that tight clothes made of noncotton fabrics can increase the risk of yeast infections as well. Another problem, says Hill, is sitting around in damp or moist clothes, like a wet bathing suit or even sweaty workout wear. To avoid problems, remove wet bathing suits as soon as possible, and change clothes immediately after you finish exercising. Then wash your genital area and dry thoroughly, if necessary using a hair dryer set on low.

You can also avoid problems by airing out your genitals after a day or a night in tight jeans or undies—by sleeping without bottoms, for example.

AN EXPERT'S OPINION ON . . .

Hot Summers and Yeast Infections

Have you noticed that you seem to get more yeast infections—and that they are harder to cure—during warm summer months? If so, you're not alone. Results of a new Canadian survey show that 48 percent of women experienced yeast infections, sometimes repeatedly, when the temperatures soar. According to gynecologist Celine Bouchard from Sainte-Foy, Quebec, heat and humidity can boost vaginal yeast infections, mostly by causing us to sweat more, which in turn makes our undergarments damp. And that, says Bouchard, is the ideal breeding ground for yeast.

weeks. If no problems occur, proceed to the next product, and so on down the line. Here, you're not only looking for a yeast infection to occur, but also any significant irritation that could signal changes in the vaginal environment. If all your products test out okay, try combining the ones you usually use together. Sometimes it's the way ingredients react to one another that causes the most irritating effects.

Risk #6—Poor bathroom hygiene: Since the intestines harbor yeast, ultimately so does stool. So any residue that makes it to your vagina following a bowel movement can introduce excess yeast into your ecosystem. And that can cause the fungus to gain control and begin growing.

Countermeasure: Always wipe from front to back, and change underwear at least once a day—more often if your panties become even a little soiled. While this makes good sense at all times, it is especially important during times when a yeast infection is already flaring or if you have had infections before.

AN EXPERT'S OPINION ON . . .

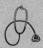

Oral Sex and Yeast Infections

Q: Can you get a yeast infection from oral sex?

A: Yes—but only if you're on the receiving end. According to a University of Michigan study on nearly 700 women, those who received oral sex twice a week or more had triple the risk of yeast infection. The reason? Up to one-third of all adults are thought to harbor the candida fungus in their mouth. Receiving oral sex from a partner who has an oral yeast infection can result in a V zone infection.

Sex and Yeast Infections

It's not considered a sexually transmitted disease—but that doesn't mean you can't get a yeast infection from having sex. Indeed, not only can you catch your initial infection from your partner, you can also get that same infection back again if you *both* resume sex after only *you* receive treatment.

While studies show that the frequency of sex-related yeast infection is highest among women who have intimate contact with other women, men *can and do* harbor yeast on their penis—with and without symptoms. When signs do appear, look for irritation, redness, and soreness on the head of his penis, sometimes accompanied by tiny white blisters.

Now if you're thinking that you can solve his problem with a few dabs of your own drugstore yeast cream, guess again. Generally men do not respond to topical treatments and instead require one of the various oral antifungal drugs. Check the section on medications later in this chapter for the drugs that work best on men.

Hormones and Yeast: Important News

Have you ever noticed that your yeast infections seem to follow a specific pattern, one that seems intimately tied to your monthly cycle? If so, your infections may be hormone related, a problem that doctors say is becoming increasingly common. How and why does this happen?

At the beginning of your cycle, estrogen levels are low. But as you head toward midcycle, they start to climb and continue to do so until ovulation occurs, around day 13 or 14.

Since the walls of your vagina contain an abundance of estrogen receptor cells, at least some of the extra hormone ends up here. Once inside the cells, however, the estrogen does not lie dormant. Instead, it begins converting other biochemicals to glycogen, a form of sugar.

Meanwhile, as soon as ovulation occurs, a second hormone known as progesterone starts to rise. As these levels climb and your period approaches, the glycogen-rich cells in the vaginal wall are shed, flooding the vaginal tissue with the sugar, which yeast loves. When sugar levels in the vagina rise, the yeast fungus can begin to grow quickly. Soon an imbalance occurs, and an infection is underway.

Once hormone levels drop, which they do just prior to the onset of bleeding, sugar levels also decline. As a result, yeast symptoms can also begin to wane. In some women, a day or two after their flow starts, nearly all symptoms are gone—only to return the following month when the hormones start to climb.

If your yeast infections follow a similar pattern, bring it to the attention of your doctor. In some cases, low-dose birth control pills may help, or your doctor may suggest a few cycles of preventative treatment with a topical antiyeast preparation beginning at midcycle.

If the cyclical infections continue, it might be prudent to have your blood sugar checked as well, with a fasting glucose tolerance test. The reason: Diabetes (see "Oreo Cookies and Yeast Infections") has also been linked to recurring yeast infections.

AN EXPERT'S OPINION ON . . .

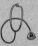

Oreo Cookies and Yeast Infections

Q: A friend told me she got a yeast infection from eating too many Oreo cookies. Can this happen?

A: It's very doubtful—unless your friend has diabetes. Here's the connection: As you just read, yeast feeds on glycogen; in fact the fungus loves it. When your body is functioning normally, your pancreas clears excess sugar from your blood, so abnormal amounts never get to your vaginal tissue. When, however, you have diabetes—a condition that causes large amounts of sugar to build in the blood—more sugar is available to feed the yeast.

According to a report by Dr. Nancy J. V. Bohannon, in the journal *Diabetes Care,* "Increased glucose levels in genital tissues enhance yeast adhesion and growth." Indeed, says Dr. Bohannon, yeast fungus cells cling to the vaginal cells of women with diabetes more readily than they do in women with normal blood sugar levels. Complicating matters further, new research shows that the failure of other mechanisms involved in regulating glucose may be linked to factors that further encourage the growth of the yeast fungus—which all goes to say that if your craving for sweets coincides with recurring yeast infections, a check for diabetes might be in order.

Pregnancy and Yeast Infections: What You Can Do

Although you might not think of pregnancy as an immunocompromised condition, in reality that's just what it is. Indeed, during gestation, your immune system is somewhat depressed, which is one reason that pregnant women are prone to a variety of vaginal infections.

Also contributing to the problem are the increased hormone levels associated with pregnancy. They too can alter your vaginal environment, further upsetting your feminine ecosystem and increasing the risk of a yeast infection.

Finally, external hemorrhoids, which frequently occur during pregnancy, can harbor yeast. Depending on exactly where they are located, the fungus could easily make its way into your vagina, further increasing the risk of a yeast infection.

The good news is that hormone levels drop dramatically after birth, and the immune system swings back into high gear. As a result, most yeast infections clear, often on their own, soon after delivery.

If, however, you want to try and clear your infection before your baby is born, never self-treat without talking to your doctor first about which medications are safest to use.

The Yeast Infection Treatment Maze: How to Get Out Alive!

Once you know for certain that a yeast infection is your V zone problem, it's time to choose your treatment regimen—no easy feat, for sure. Seven days; three days; one day. Oral; topical; natural. Prescription; over-the-counter; doctor recommended—and these are just *some* of the options from which you can choose. Indeed, many a friend has left the drugstore in tears, overwhelmed by the growing list of treatment choices. Worse still is when you think you know what will work best and it doesn't. But you keep repeating the same treatment over and over, mistakenly believing that the problem lies within your infection when it's really the product that's wrong for you.

If you've been hopelessly caught in the maze of treatment options, fear not, there is a way out—and the following treatment guide will show you the way.

Remember, however, to rely on your doctor not only for advice but also for counsel about whatever treatment you select—even an over-the-counter (OTC) preparation. In many instances, drug companies provide physicians with far more detailed information about even their OTC products than they offer to consumers, so it's likely your doctor can shed some additional light on the best ways to use the products you select.

Over the Counter and Out of the Woods

Although treatment options include both prescription and non-prescription choices, most women initially turn to OTC products first, even when their infection is diagnosed by a physician.

Despite the long and often confusing list of choices on your drugstore shelf, according to the FDA, all nonprescription antiyeast therapies are derived from a single class of drugs: the antifungal compound known as imidazole. In fact, this is the only class of medications currently approved by the FDA for the OTC treatment of yeast infection. Four versions of this basic compound are available:

- Tioconazole (sold as Vagistat, Monistat 1)
- Butoconazole (sold as Femstat 3)
- Miconazole (sold as Monistat 3 and 7)
- Clotrimazole (sold as Mycelex-7, Gyne-Lotrimin, and FemCare)

Each of these medications works in primarily the same way: by affecting the cell wall of the fungus, thus causing it to die. In terms of killing off your yeast infection, studies show that, when used properly, each of these treatments is between 85 and 90 percent effective. In addition to stomping down a yeast infection, both clotrimazole and miconazole are also used in the treatment of other skin fungus infections, including athlete's foot, jock itch, and ringworm.

Although the primary ingredients in all these treatments are chemically related, they are not identical. Additionally, each preparation has its own specific formula of inactive ingredients—things like alcohol, wax, cornstarch, and preservatives. So if you don't get relief from one product or particularly if you do get a negative reaction, such as an allergic response, you can try another with some confidence that your response will at least be different, if not better.

By the same token, the medications are not necessarily interchangeable. If you found a product to work in the past, stick with it, since using something different the next time may not necessarily give you equal results.

GOOEY THIGHS AND YEAST INFECTIONS

Q: The first time I tried a vaginal yeast product, I ended up with more on my thighs (and the bathroom floor) than I got inside. Is there a trick to getting the medication inside—and keeping it there?

A: While it's true these treatments can be messy, one way to reduce problems is to purchase products with prefilled applicators. This will at least cut down on one potentially messy step.

Next, experts say, you should stand with your legs apart and knees slightly bent. If it's more comfortable, lie down on your bed (you might want to place a towel under your buns first) with your legs spread apart and knees slightly bent. Then gently insert the applicator as far as you can without causing pain or irritation. Be certain to press the applicator plunger in *all the way.* This will help spread the cream as far into your vagina as possible. After this step is complete, you might want to wait a minute or two before pulling out the applicator, to make certain the cream has settled inside. Then *gently* remove it. If you are lying down, continue to stay in that position for a few additional minutes. If you are standing up, sit or lie down for a few minutes after removing the applicator. (These same instructions work for yeast treatments in the form of vaginal suppositories as well as vaginal insert tablets, which may also be less messy to use.)

Regardless of the type of product you choose, some medication may drip out—it's almost unavoidable. To protect panties, wear a sanitary napkin, at least for several hours following treatment. Never, however, use a tampon to keep yeast medicine inside. Not only will it absorb most of the medication, keeping it from getting into vaginal tissue, it can also cause further irritation, making your infection harder to treat.

The best time to use a yeast infection treatment is before bed-

(continued on next page)

time, particularly if you can manage to sleep on your back. Again, however, you may want to place a towel underneath you to help catch any leakage, particularly if you don't wear either panties or a sanitary napkin to bed.

Remember to avoid intercourse while using a yeast treatment, particularly if you are using condoms, a diaphragm, or a cervical cap. The chemicals in some of these products can dissolve the materials in these birth control devices.

Finally, the form the product takes—cream, suppository, or capsule—may also influence your decision about what to buy. While effectiveness is roughly the same among all three, how well a treatment works often depends on whether you use it correctly and for the correct amount of time. So, be certain to choose whichever form of treatment you are most likely to use. Often personal preferences can vary, so don't rely only on what your best friend, or sister, or mother prefers. Instead, go for what you think is best for you.

One hint: if you are used to using tampons, the prefilled applicator creams will probably work well. If you have never used a tampon, mostly because you don't like the insertion process, then these applicators may prove uncomfortable and hard to use.

One, Three, Seven: How to Choose

One of the most obvious features that separate the various anti-yeast medications is the length of the treatment itself. While in the not-too-distant past all of the products offered were seven-day regimens, today you can also select from three-day and now one-day treatments.

The important point here is that all yeast infections take seven days to clear, regardless of which medication you use. Although the number of days vary with some treatments, those that offer one- or three-day regimens are simply more potent formulas, able to continue working for several days after the treatment is administered. The shorter regimens simply limit the number of days you have to *take* your yeast treatment—not the actual length of time it takes to clear your infection.

Jumping Behind the Counter:
When Prescription Treatments Are a Must

For most women, OTC antiyeast preparations are all that's needed to bring about a cure. For some, however, a stronger, broad-spectrum antifungal becomes necessary. This can be the case when infections continually recur, or if one particularly stubborn infection won't respond to OTC products—as can sometimes occur when a yeast infection is caused by a strain other than the common *Candida albicans* fungus.

When, in fact, you do need a prescription treatment, your doctor can choose either an oral preparation, a vaginal tablet, or a cream. Here is a list of the basic choices, and what you can expect in the way of side effects.

- Fluconazole (Diflucan)—one-pill, one-dose cure.

  Side effects include skin rash, nausea or vomiting, diarrhea, stomach pain, or headache. Less commonly, look for dizziness and pallor. Blood tests may also reveal liver dysfunction or decreased potassium levels.

- Ketoconazole (Nizoral)—an oral, multi-dose pill version of the topical imidazole drugs used for OTC yeast products.

  While there are no common side effects with this drug, in rare instances it could cause sensitivity to light, menstrual irregularities, rash or itchy skin, fever or chills, dizziness or drowsiness, loss of appetite, or headache. Men can look for a temporary enlargement of breasts and temporary impotence.

- Nystatin (mycostantin vaginal)—available as either an oral tablet or a vaginal tablet.

  Oral versions may rarely cause nausea, upset stomach, and diarrhea. Vaginal products may cause irritation.

- Terconazole (Terazol 3, Terazol 7)—available as a broad-spectrum cream or vaginal suppository, both considered more potent than OTC versions.

  Common side effects are limited to headaches. Less common

TREATING YEAST INFECTIONS DURING YOUR PERIOD

One of the questions women frequently ask about yeast medications is whether they are safe to use during the menstrual cycle, a time when the gateway to the uterus is more open and any medication is more likely to make it farther into the reproductive tract. The answer is that not only are these medications safe to use during menstrual bleeding, they are often a necessity, particularly since many women find their most virulent infections flare right before or at the time their monthly bleeding begins.

Indeed, experts say that if you do experience a yeast infection just prior to or during your period, don't put off treatment until bleeding stops. Doing so could cause your infection to grow more virulent and harder to treat—even if you wait just a few days to begin.

Because using a vaginal yeast product during your period can be messier than usual, doctors suggest applying it at night, prior to bedtime. Also remember: never use a tampon for sanitary protection while you have a yeast infection.

are abdominal pain, fever, menstrual irregularities, chills, burning vagina, vaginal pain, body aches, and itching.

While all these drugs should begin to clear your infection beginning about three days after treatment, for more immediate relief of symptoms such as itching and burning, ask your doctor about an anti-inflammatory cream to use along with the oral medication. Do not, however, choose an OTC antifungal treatment cream to use along with your oral prescription unless your doctor tells you to do so.

Men who require treatment for yeast infection can choose either Diflucan or Nizoral. Since a topical vaginal preparation will not work on a penile infection, prescription drugs are the only real treatment alternatives.

Everything Old Is New Again

Predating most of the modern treatments for yeast infection was a medication known as gentian violet. As you might guess, it got its name from its bright purple color, a dye on the order of iodine, that stained not only the skin but virtually anything it touched, from sheets and towels to clothing. So although the medication worked extremely well, it was a nightmare to use and gradually went out of favor. Today it's found only in a few pharmacies, although some do special-order it for their customers.

Now, however, a new version of gentian violet has started to become available. The messy medication is now safely ensconced in a gelatin-based vaginal tablet, which gradually dissolves with your own body heat, so you get the benefits of treatment but without much of the mess. It is available as a nonprescription treatment, but talk to your doctor about whether it can help you.

In the "older-is-wiser" category is still one more treatment option: boric acid. As any urban girlfriend can tell you, not only does it kill roaches, it is a pretty swift terminator of the yeast fungus. Since it doesn't come packaged for vaginal use, if your doctor okays this treatment (and be certain to discuss it before trying), you'll have to employ a little do-it-yourself ingenuity. This will involve purchasing empty capsules from the pharmacy (size 00) and filling them with the boric acid yourself—about 600 mg total. Then insert two capsules as you would any other vaginal suppository, every night for one week. For extra prevention, you can continue to use the treatment up to twice a week for three more weeks.

How well does it work? A 1981 study published in the *American Journal of Obstetrics and Gynecology* found that boric acid capsules worked better than most other medications available at the time. This study, which treated ninety-two women with yeast infections, used the 600-mg capsules inserted into the vagina two times a day. (For long-term or chronic infections, many doctors now recommend using the capsules twice daily for up to four months.) The 1981 findings backed up two previous studies conducted in the late 1970s, which found similar results.

Mother Nature's Bounty

To treat a mild yeast infection naturally, many health experts advocate douching twice daily with an acidophilus solution. To make this, dissolve an oral acidophilus capsule containing at least 1 billion live organisms (the label will provide this information) in 10 milliliters of water. Then use any normal douche apparatus. You can also take an oral supplement internally, but this time look for products containing up to 2 billion live organisms for best results.

In addition, medical literature suggests that eating up to 8 ounces of yogurt daily (and again, it must contain active live organisms) may help. According to experts at the University of Toronto Sex Education Center, placing plain yogurt directly in your vagina is also an option, as is coating a tampon and inserting it for several hours or using yogurt capsules as a vaginal suppository. Another of their recommendations is a douche made from the herbs goldenseal and myrrh (simmer 1 tablespoon of each in 3 quarts of warm water; strain, and cool).

To offset the threat of yeast infections naturally, avoid sugar, dairy products, alcohol, aged cheeses, dried fruits, miso, melon, and peanuts. An "antiyeast tonic" suggested by many natural health experts consists of 1 teaspoon of apple cider vinegar mixed with 1 teaspoon of honey in ¼ cup of warm water, taken with each meal. Another alternative is to brew a cup of antiyeast tea consisting of two parts sage, two parts rosemary leaf, two parts mullein, and one-quarter part goldenseal root. Add 4 to 6 tablespoons of the herb mixture to 1 quart of cold water; then simmer over low heat up to 20 minutes. Strain the liquid and you've got your tea. Because it is often bitter, many women sweeten it with a little honey or cranberry juice.

Doing double duty, the tea can also be used as a douche—but not until its diluted. Here's the recipe: Combine ½ ounce of tea with 2 tablespoons of apple cider vinegar and 1 tablespoon of acidophilus culture (or ¼ cup plain yogurt) and 1 drop of tea-tree oil, with 1 quart of warm (not hot) water. Use regular douching apparatus.

In terms of herbal supplements, the editors of MotherNature .com suggest the following:

• Caprylic acid: A naturally occurring fatty acid with antibacterial properties, it is easily absorbed in the intestines, so time-released or coated supplements are best. The standard dose is 1,000 to 2,000 milligrams with meals.

• Goldenseal: The key ingredient here is berberine alkaloids, a natural type of antibacterial. In capsule form, try 250 to 500 milligrams three times a day, but use it only at periodic intervals. Otherwise you may kill off the bacteria your body needs to aid in digestion.

If you're in the kitchen, reach in your spice cabinet for oregano, peppermint, rosemary, and thyme, all of which have antifungal properties. Indeed, according to MotherNature.com, rosemary oil is a thousand times more potent than caprylic acid as a treatment against yeast. Because the herbs and the oils can cause heartburn and other symptoms in large doses, try supplements that are coated—usually 2 to 4 milligrams twice a day between meals will do the trick.

Although this is a potent treatment that works well, some women find it causes a vaginal burning and an excess of discharge for the first few days. If burning is significant or continues longer than a few days, stop treatment and call your doctor. Additionally, remember to *never take boric acid capsules by mouth*. It is a poison, and ingesting it can have disastrous results.

When Treatment Just Won't Help: What to Do

As any woman who has had a single yeast infection can tell you, once is definitely enough. However, for a growing number, the first infec-

AN EXPERT'S OPINION ON . . .

Garlic in Your Vagina

Q: I've heard that garlic is good for a yeast infection, but what do you do with it? A friend says put a clove in my vagina, but that sounds too weird. How does this treatment work?

A: Weird as it may sound, inserting the garlic into your vagina is precisely what many naturopathic physicians recommend. However, it's probably not a good idea to place the whole clove, skin and all, inside.

According to natural health expert Rosemary Gladstar, author of *Herbal Healing for Women* (New York: Fireside, 1993), the best idea is to peel a clove and then wrap it in sterile gauze, leaving a small "tail" at the end. Then insert the clove into your vagina much as you would a suppository, and leave it there for 3 to 5 hours, after which you should remove it and replace it with a fresh gauze-wrapped clove. Gladstar indicates that the treatment should be repeated several times a day for three to five days.

There are, however, a few caveats to this treatment. First, never leave a clove in your vagina for more than five hours. More important, never forget it's there altogether, leaving it for an extended period of time. Doing so can lead to a nasty infection.

Also important: if your vagina is very sensitive, be careful not to nick the clove when you peel the skin. Cutting the garlic releases more of the oils, which in turn can cause some burning. If, however, your vagina is not particularly sensitive, do make cuts in the clove, since many believe that releasing the oils will increase the curative effect on yeast infections.

In addition, according to the editors at MotherNature.com,

(continued on next page)

adding garlic to your diet may also help fight yeast infections. The key is the nutrient allicin, a powerful antibacterial agent found in garlic. Your goal should be one fresh clove per day. You can also take a garlic supplement, but it must contain at least 10 milligrams of allicin per dose (check the label for this information).

tion is just the beginning of the candida nightmare. Indeed, up to 5 percent of all women experience a recurring form of the fungus—one that not only stubbornly resists treatment but also continues to come back time and again, despite the absence of common trigger factors such as antibiotics, birth control pills, or poor hygiene habits. In fact, for these women, no discernible reason for their recurring infections can ever be found. Their infections continue without much relief, sometimes for years on end.

Traditionally, doctors believed this occurred when reserves of the candida fungus, stored naturally in the intestines, made their way to the vagina on a regular basis, where they continually worked to "reseed" the fungus supply. So no sooner was treatment for one infection completed, when more yeast was released into the vagina, and another infection began.

In a second theory called "vaginal relapse," experts contend that small colonies of fungus remain in the vagina even after treatment. Although they are too tiny to be seen, even on a slide placed under a microscope, they begin the reseeding process soon after treatment is stopped.

More recently, experts began to theorize that particularly stubborn yeast infections may be due to an allergy to the candida fungus itself. In some women it seems even the small amount of yeast found naturally in the vagina may trigger an allergic response, which in turn causes an irritation that continually leads to infection.

Although there is currently no specific treatment for recurring yeast infections, doctors say you can reduce some risks by avoiding some of the common trigger factors, such as antibiotics, whenever possible. Additionally, pay special attention to the hygiene factors that encourage yeast growth, including tight clothing.

Finally, don't try to weather recurring yeast infections on your own. See your doctor, and make certain to reveal both how long your infections have been going on and how frequently they recur. In many instances, your physician may be able to prescribe medications that can at least cut down on the number of flare-ups you experience.

HIV and Recurring Yeast Infections: The Latest News

In the early 1990s word came that recurring yeast infections, particularly those that develop without an obvious trigger factor, may be linked to HIV, the virus that causes AIDS. The report, issued by the U.S. Public Health Service, caused a panic that still leaves some women in a cold sweat.

Knowing the facts, however, should make you feel a whole lot better. Indeed, the main connection between the two diseases is that because HIV depresses the immune system, a yeast infection becomes harder to treat. As such, it can linger longer and sometimes recur more often, simply because a complete recovery never really occurs.

In addition, new evidence has begun to suggest that lactobacillus—the "good" bacteria that plummet with a yeast infection—may have some protective properties within the vagina itself, helping us to avoid contracting some sexually transmitted diseases, including HIV. Thus, when levels fall, as they do with a yeast infection, it may turn out that our risk of becoming infected soars far above normal with each and every encounter we have with an infected partner.

Clearly, for the overwhelming majority of women, there is no HIV-yeast connection. However, don't be surprised if your doctor errs on the side of caution by suggesting you take an AIDS test if and when a yeast infection seems particularly hard to cure. And certainly, it never hurts to be reassured of your overall good health by being tested.

Additionally, remember that having unprotected sex with an HIV-infected partner is a risky venture to begin with—and doing so while you have a yeast infection increases all risks, particularly if your infection has caused any open lesions inside your vagina.

Mistaken Identity: When You Think You've Got It But You Don't

For many women, no reason will ever be found for why their yeast infections recur or why common treatments don't seem to work. For some, however, the answer may simply be that they really don't have a yeast infection at all.

How can this be, particularly when the symptoms are often so obvious?

The answer comes in the form of a relatively new V zone infection known as cytolic vaginitis, a condition that so closely resembles a yeast infection (right down to its clumpy white discharge) that time and again doctors miss the diagnosis. The real problems set in, however, when patients are continually offered antiyeast therapy.

According to the *Harvard Guide to Women's Health,* not only is cytolic vaginitis a completely different condition, it also requires radically different treatment. More specifically, while a yeast infection develops out of a *deficiency* of lactobacillus bacteria and a *loss* of vaginal acid, Karen J. Carlson, M.D., Stephanie A. Eisenstat, M.D., and Terra Ziporyn, Ph.D., report that cytolic vaginitis occurs when there is a lactobacillus *overload,* resulting in a *highly acidic* environment. While normally vaginal acid is a good thing, in this instance, levels are so high that, ironically, it causes many of the same symptoms as when levels are too low, including the clumpy white discharge and the burning, itchy, red vagina, all associated with a yeast infection.

But while the goal of yeast infection treatment is to *raise* the vaginal acid level, the treatment for cytolic vaginitis concentrates on reducing it. As such, it's easy to see how making the wrong diagnosis and rendering the wrong treatment could be a real problem.

So how can you go about telling the difference between the two? You'll need your doctor's help and some laboratory procedures. These include a test of your vaginal pH, plus a smear of your vaginal secretions placed on a slide and examined under a microscope. If your vaginal pH is low (indicating high acid) and there is an abundance of lactobacillus on your slide, then it's highly likely your symptoms are the result of cytolic vaginitis, and not a yeast infection.

If this is the case, treatment is fast and easy: douching one to three times a week with a solution made from 1 to 2 ounces of baking soda to 1 quart of warm water. This reduces the acid level in your vagina, as well as the higher-than-normal levels of lactobacillus. Within a week, your vaginal environment will likely return to normal, and symptoms should subside.

Important warning: As simple as the treatment is, experts say don't be tempted to try it *without* first visiting your doctor and getting tested. If you do have a yeast infection, even one baking soda douche could cause symptoms to worsen dramatically.

Finally, if you're wondering how cytolic vaginitis occurs in the first place and where you got yours, it's doubtful you'll ever find out. This condition is so new that few details are known about how or why it occurs. The one thing that is certain, however, is that it is not sexually transmitted. So at least for now, your partner is off the hook!

A Final Word:
Self-Diagnosis vs. Medical Care

While the symptoms of a yeast infection may seem so obvious that it would be almost impossible to miss them, it can happen. Indeed, studies show that up to 67 percent of women who thought they had a yeast infection were flat-out wrong. More important, treating a yeast infection where none exists—or worse still, using an antiyeast product on a different type of infection—can have serious consequences.

That's why experts believe that initially, every first-time yeast infection should be diagnosed by a doctor—and not just over the phone. Indeed, an accurate diagnosis requires not only a first hand look at your vagina but also a laboratory test known as a "wet prep." This involves placing a drop of your vaginal secretions on a slide that contains an alkaline solution, which should dissolve everything but the fungus. Observing the slide under the microscope will show if the *Candida albicans* strain of fungus is present in larger-than-normal amounts.

If your doctor suspects your infection may be caused by one of the newer strains of *Candida,* diagnosis may also include a culture—a test that uses samples of your vaginal fluid to grow the fungus in a laboratory. Sometimes this can help identify the strain and influence treatment choices.

Once you've had your first yeast infection, however, subsequent occurrences are easier to identify, and you can feel more comfortable giving self-care a whirl. Remember, however, that your yeast infection should clear within seven days. If it doesn't or if it recurs within ten days, see your doctor right away.

CHAPTER FOUR

Itches, Rashes, Bumps, and Lumps

The V Zone Conditions You Can't Ignore

In much the same way that the skin on your hands or face or feet or tummy can become inflamed and irritated, so too can the skin and tissue covering the inside and outside of your vulva. Indeed, sometimes that inflammation can be so intense that it closely mimics symptoms caused by BV or even a yeast infection.

For most women, however, when no bacteria are present, vaginal or vulvar inflammation is the result of the chemicals, and particularly the fragrances, found in some of the most commonly used V zone products—items such as soaps, spermicides, lubricants, or hygiene sprays. All have the potential to cause a sensitivity reaction or even a true allergy, resulting in not only redness and inflammation, but a burning, itching pain that can drive you to distraction.

Medically known as vulvar vaginitis or chemical vulvitis, a sensitivity reaction can develop immediately—right after using a new product, for example—or after months or even years of trouble-free use. According to some experts, including British gynecologist Dr. Miriam Stoppard, using certain products for a long period of time can cause the vagina to become so sensitized that, at some point, you can begin to react to almost any product you use.

In addition to the products mentioned above are these other offenders:

- Laundry detergents used to wash panties or panty hose
- Detergent residues left on towels or washcloths
- Fabric softener residue
- Dry cleaning residues (particularly on tight pants)
- Bubble baths or bath gels
- Shampoo
- Condoms, particularly scented or flavored varieties
- Hair removal products
- Fragrances

Additionally, many women trace the source of their irritation to any V zone product that is scented or contains a dye, such as colored toilet paper or even certain intimate garments. Indeed, when tight-fitting panty hose first came into fashion, so many women began developing vaginal irritations that the concept of the white cotton crotch was born.

Another potential offender is sanitary protection products. While some women find that tampons can be more irritating than a sanitary

IRRITATION OR INFECTION: HOW TO TELL THE DIFFERENCE

Because many symptoms of a V zone irritation also occur in conjunction with a number of potentially serious vaginal infections, it's important that the distinction is made as early as possible. One defining factor is whether a discharge is present. Generally a discharge usually means an infection, while no discharge usually means only inflammation.

However, this is not a hard-and-fast rule. Should your cervix become involved in the inflammatory process, a condition called cervicitis, then a discharge may indeed occur, even if no infection exists. Also, remember that sometimes both an inflammation and an infection can occur simultaneously.

napkin, as both the source of inflammation and as a contributing factor, others find the new moisture-resistant covers on pads to be even more problematic. The inflammatory potential of either product increases even further when it contains fragrance or deodorant.

Discovering Your Source of Trouble: What to Do

Among the best ways to reduce irritating V zone symptoms is to find the source of your problem. Experts say the best place to start is by eliminating all unessential products that come in contact with your V zone, particularly bubble bath, shower gels, dusting powder, deodorant sprays, lubricants, and any scented or colored product. If problems don't clear within seven to ten days, look to more subtle causes such as laundry detergent, fabric softener, panty liners, or even your panties or panty hose.

If your inflammation begins to clear after eliminating one specific product, then it was likely the cause of your irritation. If, however, you are like most other women, you probably eliminated a whole bunch of products all at once. If this is the case and your inflammation clears, you will have to take an extra step to determine just what was the cause.

This will involve reintroducing your V zone to each potential offender, *one product at a time,* using each one by itself for one to two weeks. If you remain irritation free, stop using it, and move on to the next product.

If, after trying all the items, you still remain irritation free, it's possible your symptoms may have been the result of the combined ingredients of two or more products, such as a spermicide and a condom or a sanitary napkin and a deodorant spray. To find out, begin trying two products at a time, selecting those that you normally used within twelve hours of each other. Again, take at least two weeks per combination, and watch your V zone for signs of trouble. In most instances the irritation will recur in direct response to a particular combination.

Taking the Cure

For many women, locating the source of the problem and eliminating it is all that's necessary to bring about a cure. For others, inflammation can be so intense that even discontinuing the offending product won't bring relief. When this is the case, one of several anti-inflammatory creams or lotions may help—usually those containing at least 1 percent hydrocortisone.

Be aware, however, that when V zone tissue is already sensitized and irritated, some extra ingredients found in these products, like base creams, can cause problems. If, despite your best efforts, irritations continue, talk to your doctor about which prescription medications can help.

The Hour-Glass Irritation: What to Look For

For most women, V zone irritations spread randomly throughout the vulva, with no particular pattern to either the redness or the irritation. Sometimes, however, specific problems can be identified by the precise pattern with which they do occur. One of the most common is called *lichen sclerosus*. A chronic skin disorder, according to experts at the University of Michigan Center for Vulvar Diseases, its main symptom is itching, accompanied by inflammation occurring in a distinct hour-glass shape, starting from the clitoris, spreading out into the labia, and then outward toward the anus. Within this shape there will be ivory-colored patches, often surrounded by pink, inflamed skin. Further, V zone tissue can become rough and dry and take on an almost parchment-like appearance (some women say it resembles a crinkled cigarette paper). As time goes by, the skin can become thickened, taking on a rough, weathered appearance that is often accompanied by vulvar pain and itching. In some instances, the itching can become so intense and the skin so inflamed that it actually splits, causing small, painful tears within the inner folds of the labia. Although it does not spread into the vagina, in some women the opening can become so eroded that intercourse becomes painful and difficult. Indeed, for many women, lichen sclerosus leads to vulvar vestibulitis (see Chapter 5), a chronic type of vulvar pain that can make intercourse difficult or even impossible.

Although the symptoms make lichen sclerosus easy to spot, in many instances you will need a colposcopy (a special X ray) or a biopsy to confirm the diagnosis. This will rule out the very small possibility that your symptoms could be early signs of vulvar cancer.

AN EXPERT'S OPINION ON . . .

Avoiding V Zone Irritations: What to Do

- Use only white, unscented toilet tissue.
- If a need for sanitary protection products turns out to be the source of your problems, look for all-cotton pads and tampons. (See "Resources for Better Health.")
- Use unscented soaps, and when possible avoid all commercial soaps, opting instead for those found at body and bath shops, or in specialty catalogs.
- Wear cotton underwear, preferably white, particularly while the irritation is flaring.
- Wash your V zone every day, and make certain to dry it thoroughly .
- Avoid all scented V zone products, and *don't* spray your regular cologne or perfume on your panties, panty liners, or sanitary pads or tampons.
- Sleep without a bottom.
- Change out of wet bathing suits or sweaty workout clothes as soon as possible.
- Avoid V zone products containing alpha hydroxy acids, dye, alcohol, or propylene glycol.

Source: Adapted from the Vulvar Pain Foundation Guidelines.

Once lichen sclerosus is diagnosed, treatment can help. The goal is to eliminate itching and protect the skin from further damage, which in the past was accomplished with prescription testosterone cream. Now, doctors at the Michigan Center for Vulvar Diseases report that many physicians are now turning to a topical steroid instead, particularly a prescription cream known as clobetasol. Switching to a mild, nonirritating soap for cleansing, and avoiding tight-fitting clothes during treatment, can also help. In extreme cases, surgery may be necessary for symptom relief.

Are You At Risk? How to Tell

Although most often lichen sclerosus occurs after menopause, it can develop any time during a woman's life. Younger women often find it develops more readily directly after pregnancy. While no one is certain why it occurs, some research has shown the cause may have a genetic link. According to experts at the University of Iowa Women's Health Center, there may also be an immune component as well. Here, antibodies that normally help the body fight infection instead begin attacking the skin.

IMPORTANT WARNING

For most women, early treatment of lichen sclerosus brings about a complete cure, with little risk of recurrence. If left untreated long enough, however, V zone scar tissue can result, a problem that can lead to a localized skin cancer. Although the risk of cancer is quite small—it occurs in fewer than 10 percent of patients—if scar tissue does develop, your vulva must be examined regularly by your gynecologist.

Additionally, if you develop any V zone sores or ulcers that last longer than a few weeks, lesions that bleed easily, or bumps or raised lesions that grow rapidly within a few weeks, see your gynecologist right away. While it's not likely to be a serious problem, catching any condition at its earliest stage increases your chances for a quick and complete recovery.

Mother Nature's Bounty

In addition to whatever products you may find on your drugstore shelf, many women report a number of natural ingredients as being helpful for vaginal or vulvar irritations.

Among the most popular is a homemade natural clay powder, which is reportedly extremely effective in soothing an irritating, itchy, red rash. The recipe consists of 1 cup of fine white clay (available in most health food stores) combined with ½ cup cornstarch, 2 tablespoons of black walnut powder, 2 tablespoons of myrrh, and 1 tablespoon of goldenseal powder. Sift together and place in a glass jar. To use, shake out a small amount on a body dusting brush, and apply to the outside of your vagina and partway to the inner lips.

One of the most soothing of all herbs for any skin irritation is calendula flowers. You can also make your own calendula preparations by mixing 1 part of these dried flowers with 1 part St. John's wort flower and 1 part comfrey leaves. Cover the mixture with a high-quality vegetable oil (such as olive or walnut), and place it in a double boiler for 30 to 60 minutes. The lower the heat and the longer you cook them, the better it is. Strain the oil and add ¼ cup beeswax to the mixture, and heat again over low flame until the wax melts. For a softer, easier-to-spread balm, add more oil and less beeswax; for a firm salve, add more beeswax. When the mixture cools, apply liberally to vaginal tissue as needed. Pour the remainder into a glass jar, and store in a cool, dark place for up to one year.

The one thing everyone is sure of, however, is that lichen sclerosus is *not infectious.* You can't get it from anyone else, and you can't spread it.

When Your V Zone
Goes Bump in the Night

You go to bed, and everything is fine. But you wake up to discover a series of tiny, itchy white bumps on the inside or the outside of your V zone. So closely resembling premenstrual breakouts on the face, many women wonder whether they have developed a bizarre case of vaginal acne!

In reality, however, the problem is an exotic-sounding but all-too-common condition known as *lichen planus,* a noninfectious skin inflammation that can occur not only on the genitals but also on the shins, wrist, and hands. While no one is certain how or why it occurs, if left untreated, the surrounding skin can become so inflamed and painful that great discomfort results. In some instances scar tissue may even develop.

Although most gynecologists recognize lichen planus on sight, it does require a biopsy for accurate diagnosis. Once confirmed, it can be easily treated with a variety of prescription creams and ointments—preparations that will relieve the itching and redness and clear away the bumps.

Although you may be able to self-treat lichen planus symptoms using over-the-counter steroid creams, you should still have your diagnosis confirmed by a doctor. The reason: though the risk is small, there is a tiny chance this condition can also progress to a localized vulvar cancer, something your doctor can quickly and easily rule out.

Lumps, Bumps, and Swollen Glands

Perhaps nothing else throws a woman more off balance than to glance down at her V zone and spot a round, bulging growth, particularly if it's tender to the touch. While for many, the first thought is "tumor," for the overwhelming majority the diagnosis will be a cyst—a liquid or semisolid filled sac that can develop almost anywhere in the V zone. Among the most common sites are the Bartholin's glands—tiny, pea-sized mucus-secreting organs that lie on either side of your vaginal opening. Normally you wouldn't even notice they are there. But when something obstructs their secretory function (such as an infection or even a trauma to the vagina), the mucus becomes plugged inside the gland. Soon afterward, the gland itself becomes inflamed and the cyst forms, sometimes growing as large as 1 or 2 inches in size (see illustration).

Although it can be painful, if you are under age forty, your doctor

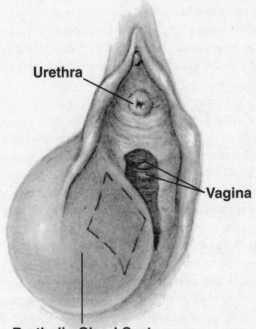

Urethra

Vagina

Bartholin Gland Cyst

BARTHOLIN GLAND CYST

Developing on the outer portion of the vagina, a Bartholin Gland cyst can be as small as a peanut or as large as a lemon. In many instances it will disappear on its own. When surgery is necessary, a small diamond-shaped incision is made on the surface of the cyst and the growth is removed.

Courtesy of Lippincott, Williams & Wilkins, Medi-Clip

may suggest simply leaving it alone. Most often, the cyst will disappear on its own, particularly if you avoid wearing tight jeans and undies for about ten days. However, according to the Academy of Family Physicians, if the gland becomes painful, particularly when walking or during intercourse or if the cyst becomes red, inflamed, hot, or tender, you may also have developed an abscess within the gland. This is an infection that, if left untreated, can spread within your entire V zone. In this case, Academy guidelines suggest antibiotics to help clear the infection, as well as one or more surgical interventions to help drain the gland. In most instances it can done in your doctor's office using local anesthesia.

If the cyst continues to recur (a rare occurrence) your doctor may suggest a slightly more complex draining procedure known as *marsupialization*. In a very small number of women (primarily those over age forty), the entire gland will be removed and biopsied for a rare form of cancer.

Other V Zone Cysts

In addition to the Bartholin gland cysts, other types of V zone growths can develop as well. Among the most common results when a hair follicle grows inward, causing a fluid-filled sac to develop. Often resembling a boil, they can range in size from ⅛ inch to over 1 inch in diameter and are often tender to the touch. Usually, however, they don't require much in the way of medical treatment. Normally hot, moist compresses can help relieve the inflammation and allow the sac to drain on its own.

Some women also develop what are known as sebaceous, or oil-filled cysts in their V zone. Soft and smooth to the touch, they can appear yellowish in color—usually the result of the oily fluid on the inside.

Although neither cyst represents a major health threat, they should be diagnosed by your doctor, who will usually extract a small amount of fluid for lab analysis. This will help rule out the threat of any serious infection.

Do not attempt to squeeze or in any way aspirate fluid from your own V zone cyst. Doing so can introduce bacteria that can turn an otherwise harmless lump into a raging infection, which may require the cyst to be opened and surgically drained.

Intimate Lesions You Can't Ignore

For most women, V zone inflammations are benign and usually harmless. For a few, however, they can represent a more serious health threat. This is the case when your inflammation is caused by a condition known as vulvar intraepithelial neoplasm, or VIN. According to the Center for Vulvar Disease, VIN is a precancerous condition that occurs when changes in the cells of the vulvar tissue cause abnormal growth, increasing the risk of malignancy.

The good news is that even when cancer cells are present, the growth is extremely slow, meaning there is lots of time to diagnose and treat the condition before any life-threatening consequences develop.

Complicating matters just a bit, however, is that the very obvious symptoms, such as itching or burning, aren't always present. Sometimes all you might find are raised brown, pink, or white lesions on the inside of your vulva—but only if you actively look for them. That's one reason that many doctors now recommend you perform a vulvar self-exam (see Chapter 1) as often as you do a self-breast check—at least once a month.

If you do notice the characteristic lesions, diagnosis usually requires a biopsy. If VIN is confirmed, experts at the University of Iowa Women's Health Center report that treatment choices include topical preparations such as 1 percent fluorouracil cream, which helps remove the abnormal cells so new, healthy cells can grow; injections of the immune stimulant interferon, which helps the body fight the growth of abnormal cells; and surgical or laser removal of the abnormal cells.

Although the treatments can be successful, follow-up care is essential, since, say the experts, VIN can recur.

Women of any age can develop VIN, but there appears to be an increase in the number of younger women diagnosed with this condition. Risk factors include fair skin, genital warts, smoking, and any condition that compromises the immune system. Some forms of VIN may also be sexually transmitted.

Avoiding Vulvar Cancer:
What You Must Do

Far less serious than VIN but still worthy of your concern is a condition known as squamous cell hyperplasia—in simple terms, an overgrowth of skin cell tissues within the vulva. Although it is far less likely to lead to vulvar cancer than VIN, it *can* happen—and for that reason you should become familiar with the symptoms.

The most obvious, and usually the earliest, sign is a bright pink or red vulva. It can also appear as elevated white patches in irregular shapes. The size of the patches can range from very small—about the size of a pea—to quite extensive. Most often they are seen on the hood of the clitoris, plus the inside and outside lips of the vulva. Sometimes they extend downward to the top of the thighs.

According to the Center for Vulvar Diseases, as the condition progresses, the vulvar skin will become thicker and harder, mostly in response to the irritation. Moisture, scratching, or washing with a rough cloth can alter the appearance of the lesions, making them look more prominent and redder in color.

To diagnose squamous cell hyperplasia, your doctor will need to perform a biopsy, particularly since it sometimes can be observed next to invasive squamous cell cancer. However, it's important to note that on its own, squamous cell hyperplasia very rarely becomes malignant. Indeed, as long as no cancer is diagnosed (the case for the majority of women) long-term use of steroid creams is the only treatment necessary.

A Final Word

Although almost any V zone inflammation can cause you worry and fear, the truth is that very few of these problems lead to serious health threats, particularly when diagnosed early on.

That said, it is not wise to ignore any abnormal vulvar symptoms, particularly redness, itching, and irritation. Although it's always best to see your doctor *before* trying self-care, if you are like most other women, you are likely to run to the drugstore before you go to the gynecologist. If so, make certain to see your doctor if symptoms last longer than seven days—or certainly if they grow worse with self-care. And if you develop a fever or any flulike symptoms during treatment, call your doctor right away.

CHAPTER FIVE

The Mysterious V Pain Syndrome

What Every Woman Needs to Know

It has been described as a constant throbbing, or sometimes a burning, searing raw irritation that extends anywhere from the outside of the vulva clear to the inside of the vagina—and even down to the thighs and the lower body. For some women, it is most intense when pressure is applied—during intercourse, for example, or when inserting a tampon. For others, simply wearing slacks or tight-fitting underwear sends shock waves through their entire pelvic region.

The problem is medically known as *vulvodynia,* a unique form of vulvar pain that is said to affect at least 15 percent of all women, mostly beginning at around age twenty-five. According to the Vulvar Pain Foundation, young white women are by far the most likely to be affected, but it can strike any woman, at any age.

Unfortunately, however, even in this more enlightened age of women's health care, many doctors remain in the dark about vulvar pain, which is one reason that experts consider it the most commonly misdiagnosed problem in gynecology. "Because of a lack of awareness of this condition, positive interventions are often not offered," says Dr. William Ledger, chairman of the Department of Obstetrics and Gynecology at New York Presbyterian Hospital–Cornell Medical Center.

But as any woman who has experienced vulvodynia can tell you, the problem *is* pretty hard to miss. So how come something so obvious has gone untreated for so long?

One answer lies in the fact that until fairly recently, the problem itself didn't even have a medical name.

Sex, Medicine, and Women's Rights

The idea that a woman can experience vulvar pain is certainly not new. Indeed, doctors have long known it can develop as a result of any number of problems, from sexually transmitted diseases, to vaginal infections, physical trauma to the genitals, or even an allergic reaction to intimate products or clothing such as panties or panty hose. Autoimmune diseases such as lupus and Crohn's disease can cause painful lesions on the vulva and vagina, and pain can result from a blocked or inflamed Bartholin's gland (see Chapter 4). Certainly, intercourse can be difficult when any of these conditions exist.

However, when it came to vulvar pain that occurred *independently* of any known disorder, medical science continually came up short. Although the concept was first documented in 1889 (doctors described it as "excessive sensitivity of the nerves supplying the mucous membrane") and then again later in the 1930s, it wasn't until 1975 that the term *vulvodynia* even appeared in medical literature—and even then it took us only halfway there. Indeed, the term was expanded to encompass *any and all* vulvar pain, particularly that which was caused by infections, such as BV or yeast.

Under those circumstances, women who continued to complain of *unexplained* vulvar pain, particularly during intercourse, were still being dismissed as "hysterical." Often diagnosed as channeling anxieties and fears into physical complaints, they were usually sent home with a pat on the head and a prescription for tranquilizers.

And so it went until 1987. That's when American gynecologist Dr. Edward Friedrich categorized an important subgroup of vulvar pain. He named the condition *vulvar vestibulitis* and defined it as moderate to severe pain when a particular section of the vulva (called the vestibule) was even lightly touched. More important, his research documented that *vulvar pain could exist in the absence of any discernible cause.*

By 1991, a second researcher, Clive C. Solomons, Ph.D., the former director of research at the University of Colorado Health Sciences Center in Denver, made another significant contribution by publishing the first medical case study to document unexplained vulvar pain.

But despite efforts by these and other experts, as recently as 1992 the *Merck Manual,* the ultimate diagnostic reference guide for physicians, still continued to list vulvar pain during intercourse under "Psychiatric Disturbances." Nowhere in the index was there even a mention of the terms *vulvodynia* or *vulvar vestibulitis.*

In fact, it wasn't until women themselves took matters into their own hands that things really began to change. In the early 1990s an important grass-roots organization came together as the Vulvar Pain Foundation, a collaboration between patients and a few physicians dedicated to spreading the word about this grossly neglected women's health problem. It wasn't long before other groups began springing up as well, including the National Vulvodynia Association and the Vulvar Pain Foundation. (See "Resources for Better Health.") By 1997, the National Institutes of Health convened a special investigative panel with a single purpose: to gather research about vulvodynia.

Today there is a rapidly growing number of doctors and researchers who not only believe that vulvar pain can exist independent of any infection or disease, they are continually developing treatments to help ease that pain. By some estimates, more than 80 percent of women who suffer with this debilitating condition can now find significant relief.

So, why does vulvodynia *still* remain one of the most misdiagnosed problems in women's health care? Even today, many doctors still remain in the dark about this subject. Some are so unfamiliar with treatment options that they subject women to expensive, painful, and sometimes damaging care. Others continue to label patients as "frigid" or suggest they explore a different sexual orientation.

The important point to remember, however, is that *none of this need be true for you.* If you suffer from vulvar pain there *are* experts who can help and treatments that really do work. But before you learn what you can do about your problem, it's important that you understand a little something about how and why vulvodynia occurs and the triggers that might be igniting your pain.

Making Love, Tight Jeans, and Vulvar Pain: Important Connections

If you have even the slightest knowledge about how your body works, it will come as no surprise that many experts continue to cite sex as the main trigger for vulvodynia. Indeed, from strictly a biological point of view, being the recipient of intense penile thrusting, as well as assuming the various back, leg, and hip movements involved in making love, it's clear a woman's role as a sexual partner is no easy feat. Additionally, the vulva, a network of delicate nerve endings that increase your sexual pleasure, becomes the focus of some pretty intense pressure during sex. So, should something in that network go wrong, it's not hard to see how pleasure can quickly turn to pain.

That said, many women also report that a wide variety of situations can trigger vulvar pain—everything from wearing tight jeans and underwear, to sanitary napkins, to sitting in certain positions, playing sports, or sometimes even just walking up a flight of stairs. For some, the pain is constant; for others, it's chronic but cyclical. While many do have extreme difficulty with intercourse, for others activities such as bike riding are far worse to endure.

What Causes V Zone Pain: The Latest News

Although experts once sought to find a single factor causing vulvar pain symptoms in all women, we now know this likely is not the case. Indeed, experts have identified at least three different subcategories of vulvar pain, and each appears to have its own subset of causes.

If you do experience vulvar pain, your doctor may classify your problem using one of the following three categories:

Cyclical vulvovaginitis. Pain usually grows worse just before or during the menstrual cycle and can be particularly intense during intercourse as well as the day after. Often there are symptom-free days as well. Many women who have this type of vulvar pain often have a hypersensitivity to the *Candida* fungus.

Vulvar vestibulitis. There is tenderness and pain when particular areas of the vulva are even lightly touched, making intercourse very painful. Pain can be intermittent or cyclical. According to a recent report in the *Journal of Women's Health,* vulvar vestibulitis is most common among young white women, particularly those who have experienced recurring yeast infections—perhaps due to the chronic irritation or overuse of certain medications. Causes of this type of vulvar pain can include chemical sensitivities or other irritants, a history of laser surgery or cryotherapy, or an allergic drug reaction. More recently some studies have suggested links to a previously undiagnosed infection with the human papilloma virus (HPV) (see Chapter 8).

Dyesthetic vulvodynia. Also known as *essential vulvodynia,* the hallmark here is unrelenting vulvar burning that rarely subsides. There is often some pain on intercourse, but many women find they can tolerate sex some of the time. The onset usually occurs after age forty-five and is sometimes misdiagnosed as vaginal dryness due to a decrease in estrogen levels associated with menopause. Often the problem is rooted in neurological causes.

Most recently, researchers have identified specific cytokines (substances released by cells and linked to pain and inflammation) present in the vulvar skin of some vulvodynia patients—cells that may be responsible for some of the pain associated with any of the three categories of vulvar pain. According to the National Vulvar Association, pain can also be associated with physical trauma to the vagina (sometimes the result of sex aids or rough sex). Sometimes it begins after childbirth, owing to certain physiological traumas occurring during labor and delivery, or following a yeast infection.

Pain can also be the result of spasms in the muscles that support the pelvic organs or because of higher-than-normal urinary levels of a natural chemical called oxalate crystals, a by-product that forms when certain foods are eaten—particularly chocolate, beer, tea, and citrus fruits. (See "The Low-Oxalate Diet Foods" later in this chapter.)

AN EXPERT'S OPINION ON . . .

Vulvodynia—Could You Have It?
How to Tell

Although pain during intercourse is one clue that vulvodynia may be your problem, vulvar pain can occur almost anytime, in any situation. According to the International Society for the Study of Vulvovaginal Disease, you can also look for these symptoms:

- Intense irritation
- Rawness
- Burning
- Stinging
- Shooting pains in the vulva or vagina
- Hypersensitivity
- Swelling of the vulva
- Rectal itching and burning
- Frequent, sometimes painful bowel movements.

For many, symptoms are also accompanied by urological complaints:

- Urgency and frequency of urination
- Bladder or urethral burning
- Blood in the urine, even when no infection is present
- Increased incidence of interstitial cystitis (see Chapter 6).

According to the National Vulvodynia Association (NVA), 35 percent of women with vulvar pain also have symptoms of fibromyalgia, an autoimmune disorder that causes chronic fatigue and painful muscles and joints. Indeed, many women say that their V zone pain occurs in conjunction with a host of full-body symptoms, including headaches, allergies, chemical sensitivities, and burning mouth and tongue. The NVA also reports that up to 50 percent of vulvar pain patients experience irritable bowel syndrome.

Diagnosing *Your* V Zone Pain: What Your Doctor Can Do

One of the most frustrating aspects of accurately diagnosing vulvar pain is that other than the pain itself, for many women there may be few, if any other, symptoms, particularly if no secondary infection or trauma is present. Although sometimes the vulva may appear slightly redder than usual or have microscopic paper cuts, it may look totally normal unless the tissue is examined under a powerful microscope.

What can help speed the diagnosis, however, is an adequate medical history. While this is an important part of any exam, experts who treat vulvodynia say that it is *the* most crucial part of your vulvar pain examination. Generally your doctor will need the following information:

- When your pain first began
- If any significant event occurred just prior to the pain, such as childbirth, gynecological surgery, a vaginal infection, any illness requiring you to take antibiotics, or any injury or trauma to the vulvar area
- If you regularly spend two or more hours per week on a stationary or regular bicycle
- Any specific activities that trigger your pain, such as intercourse, inserting a tampon, walking up stairs, exercising, or sitting
- The duration of your pain, including when it crests or peaks
- The existence of any urinary symptoms, particularly urgency
- If your pain is constant or if it occurs in cycles—for example, just prior to a menstrual period
- If any close female member of your family has suffered similar pain

Try to be as precise as you can in describing how you feel, including the description of your pain (burning, throbbing, raw, irritated), where it occurs, as well as whether it spreads to other parts of your body, including your thighs, lower stomach, buttocks, or even your feet or back.

TALKING POINT

While there are many physicians who are experts in the treatment of vulvar pain, still, many doctors are not as familiar with this problem as perhaps they ought to be. Old attitudes certainly die hard, particularly in regard to women's health.

If you are suffering vulvar pain, you need to find a doctor who is on top of this problem and savvy about the latest treatment options. To gauge your doctor's expertise, ask how many vulvar pain patients he or she has treated and request the chance to speak to one or two before you accept treatment.

If you don't feel comfortable being this bold, simply ask your doctor what the latest treatments are for vulvar pain. If he or she doesn't mention at least some of the information in this chapter, then you should consider seeking a second opinion before being treated.

The "Q Tip Test"

While your doctor certainly should not doubt the existence of your pain, it is important that the description of your symptoms be accurate. For this reason, he or she may test your vulvar pain threshold, a way of determining not only how painful your condition is, but also the precise areas of your vulva that are the most sensitive. The exam is known as the "Q tip test" because your doctor often uses a long, thin swab to touch and press various areas of your vulva, looking for specific trigger points.

Testing for Infection

Often vulvar pain can be the result of an intimate infection—a sexually transmitted disease, for example, or a form of vaginitis. For a thorough diagnosis of your pain, your doctor should not only examine your vulva for outward signs of disease but also gather samples of vaginal fluids and sometimes take a snippet of tissue to biopsy for cell changes. Also important is a pH (acid) level test of your vagina, as well as certain urine analysis, particularly a twenty-four-hour test that measures levels of oxalate crystal. Why are all these tests so important? Symptoms of vulvar vestibulitis can often overlap with those of a yeast infection. According to studies conducted by Dr. Ledger and published in *Infectious Diseases in Obstetrics and Gynecology,* as a result the tendency to overdiagnose this infection is great. Even when discharge was present, reports Ledger, diagnostic evaluations of women with vulvar pain, including either a vaginal fluid test or a culture for yeast and bacteria, yielded only a 14.5 percent occurrence of yeast infection. However, in 24.1 percent of cases, the studies showed the presence of human papilloma virus (see Chapter 8), and in 19.5 percent of cases, allergic vaginitis was diagnosed. Still, more than 36 percent of the women showed no clear, recognizable cause for their vulvar pain. Under such circumstances, it's vital that any tests for infection be thorough before a diagnosis of your pain is made.

INFECTIONS THAT CAUSE VULVAR PAIN

- Herpes
- HPV—genital warts
- Yeast infection
- Lichen sclerosis
- Lichen planus
- Gonorrhea
- Neoplastic vulvar lesions
- Bacterial vaginosis

Check the index for where to find more information on these infections elsewhere in this book.

In addition, vulvar pain can result from chemical irritations caused by laundry detergents, fabric dyes, sanitary napkins, tampons, deodorant sprays, lubricants, spermicides, or condoms. Among the most irritating ingredients are propylene glycol, alcohol, dyes, and fragrance.

Muscle Tone and Vulvar Pain

Because tension in the pelvis can contribute to vulvar pain, specialists in treating vulvodynia often suggest your exam include an assessment of pelvic floor muscles, the structure that helps hold your reproductive organs in place. To test muscle tone, your doctor will manually examine your pelvis and may also use a diagnostic procedure called *electromyography,* a way of electronically "reading" muscle tension. Relatively painless, the test involves inserting a small sensor into your vagina able to detect pelvic muscle activity. The sensor then sends signals back to a small computer, which analyzes the data.

Devising Your Treatment Plan

Once your doctor determines a variety of specifics about your vulvar pain, including possible causes, there are a number of treatments that can help. Certainly the first and easiest line of defense is to treat any obvious problems, such as a yeast infection or an injury to the genitals, as well as to remove the threat of any potential allergens, such as intimate care products or even the laundry soap used to wash your lingerie (see Chapter 9).

If problems persist, you may be a candidate for any number of slightly more complex treatment options. Although not all of them will work for all women, and some will require more than one method be used simultaneously, experts have found that significant relief is possible in almost all cases of vulvodynia. However, it's important to note that nearly all treatments require a minimum of three months, and usually longer, before any substantial results are seen. For those who do stick with the various regimens, however, relief is often long-lasting and sometimes permanent.

There is also one caveat to keep in mind when reviewing your treatment options. Although many of the suggestions you will find here can be done in the self-care mode, experts caution against self-treatment for vulvar pain. Indeed, because the reactions to the treatments can be so personal and, in fact, the symptoms themselves often highly individualized, success is much more likely when you are under the care of an expert who can regularly monitor your progress.

The Diet That Makes a Difference

It has long been known that oxalate, a natural substance found in varying amounts in all plant foods, can cause various types of tissue inflammation in some people. For more than twenty years, diets that limit the intake of high-oxalate foods have been used to reduce the risk of kidney stones, as well as other renal disorders. Colorado researcher Clive Solomons, Ph.D., theorized that perhaps limiting oxalate foods in women with vulvar pain could reduce inflammation here as well. To help put his theories to the test, Solomons launched a decade-long research project involving some 2,000 women diagnosed with vulvodynia.

The study, appropriately called the Pain Project, began with urine tests to see if these patients were excreting larger-than-normal amounts of oxalate, an indication that they were sensitive to this substance. The next step was to correlate the oxalate surges found in the urine with vulvar pain symptoms. Indeed, Solomons found that the incidence of vulvar pain, as well as episodes of urinary frequency and urgency, rectal itching and burning, irritable bowel, muscle and joint pain, and burning of the mouth and tongue did, indeed, coincide *with high levels of oxalate secretion in the urine.* Not surprisingly, when oxalate levels dropped, symptoms subsided.

The next step was to see if diet could make a difference. Since foods were already categorized by oxalate content—low, medium, and high—Solomons asked the women to follow an eating plan focused on low-oxalate meals for at least several weeks. Only after symptoms improved were they advised to add foods from the other two categories.

The end result: After just several weeks on the low-oxalate diet, symptoms *did* begin to clear. According to Solomons' research, low-oxalate foods *did* make a difference, and a new treatment option was born.

It's important to note that although Dr. Solomons' work has reportedly helped thousands of women overcome vulvar pain, his studies have not been conducted under strict scientific conditions, a fact for which he has received some harsh criticism. And at least one other study disputes his findings, showing through research that women with vulvar pain do not necessarily excrete higher-than-normal levels of oxalate crystals.

But it's also important to note that many top medical leaders believe his concepts are sound and his treatment suggestions can and do work. In studies conducted at New York Hospital–Cornell Medical Center, 14.3 percent of 220 women diagnosed with vulvar vestibulitis were helped by a low oxalate diet and calcium citrate supplements. So if you want to give it a try, a low-oxalate cookbook is available from the Vulvar Pain Foundation. (See "Resources for Better Health.") You can also formulate your own diet based on the food list included in this chapter. (See "The Low-Oxalate Diet Foods.")

Nutritional Supplements That Can Help

In addition to the oxalate diet, women in the Pain Project were also encouraged to use two nutritional supplements. The first, *calcium citrate,* is a form of the mineral calcium that has a chemical structure similar to oxalate. Thus, it competes for the same place within vulvar tissue. The only difference here is that calcium citrate does not cause the same type of irritating symptoms as the oxalate. Solomons' theory held that the more calcium citrate there was in tissues, the less room there would be for oxalic acid, which in turn would reduce vulvar pain.

Again, the Pain Project proved him right. When used in conjunction with a low-oxalate diet, over time (usually three months to a year) calcium citrate reduced vulvar pain in up to 70 percent of the women in the study. In further studies, it was shown that when calcium citrate was taken in advance of the expected oxalate urine surges, up to 66 percent more of the women were able to reduce their pain, over and above those who took it randomly.

Calcium citrate supplements are readily available in most health food stores, but it may take a little detective work on your part to end up with the right product. The reason is that products will likely be labeled simply as calcium. It's not until you read the actual source label on the back of the bottle that you will find the form of calcium used. In this case, you are obviously looking for the words *calcium citrate* on that label.

In addition, there is also one caveat concerning this supplement: No one dosage is right for every woman. Additionally, even slight variations can increase or decrease pain depending on the stage of treatment. Again, it's a good idea for your treatment to be monitored by a physician familiar with this therapy.

The second supplement found to have an impact was an amino acid sugar known as *N-acetyl-glucosamine (NAG)*. Sold only in more sophisticated health food stores (usually packaged under the ingredient name NAG), it works, say experts, by increasing levels of hyaluronic acid, a substance that helps protect nerves and skin. How can this help? When, due to any number of biochemical forces, hyaluronic acid levels drop too low, tissue begins to thin, and ultimately inflammation develops. When that tissue is in the vulva, vulvodynia can result. Conversely, by boosting production of hyaluronic acid and ensuring levels remain high, NAG supplements may stop pain before it starts.

Indeed, Pain Project studies conducted in May 1997 revealed that 58 percent of some 550 participants who added NAG to their low oxalate/calcium citrate regimen for just four months significantly decreased vulvar pain over those who tried diet intervention alone.

One important point: Don't confuse this form of glucosamine with the popular pain and arthritis supplement glucosamine sulfate, now being widely sold. While sometimes NAG is included in these products (they are often packaged together), unless the label specifically says the product contains N-acetyl-glucosamine, it won't help you.

More Nutritional Supplements That Can Help

While research on the role of supplements in the treatment of vulvar pain is limited, many women report success using the following natural treatments:

- Biotin—may reduce redness and itching
- Grape seed extract—may help heal damaged tissue (but could temporarily increase urinary burning)

- L-arginine—an amino acid that may help calm urethral spasms (do not use if you have genital herpes)
- Vitamins A and E—may reduce inflammation and itching

THE LOW-OXALATE DIET FOODS

According to the *Low Oxalate Cookbook* published by the Vulvar Pain Foundation, here are some of the most common low-oxalate foods, as well as the high-oxalate ones you should avoid.

Beverages
Low oxalate: Cider; colas; fruit juices including apple, grapefruit, lemon, lime, pineapple; ginger ale; lemonade; root beer; water; red wine; herbal teas in cranberry, apple, chamomile, and peppermint flavors
Avoid: Beer, chocolate milk, cocoa, berry juices, Ovaltine, black tea, and herbal teas in lemon, orange spice, peach, and strawberry

Dairy
Low oxalate: Butter, buttermilk, cheese, milk, yogurt
Avoid: None

Fruits
Low oxalate: Apples, avocado, cherries, cranberries, seedless green grapes, lemons, mangoes, melons, nectarines, papaya, raisins
Avoid: Blackberries, blueberries, red currants, concord grapes, figs, kiwi, lemon peel, lime peel, orange peel, raspberries, strawberries, tangerines

Grains
Low oxalate: Cornflakes, egg noodles, white rice, wild rice, rye bread

(continued on next page)

Avoid: Whole wheat bread, Cheerios, graham crackers, graham flour, grits, oatmeal, popcorn, soybean crackers, spelt, stone ground flour, wheat bran, wheat germ, whole wheat flour

Meats
Low oxalate: Bacon, beef, chicken, corned beef, eggs, fish (haddock, plaice, flounder), ham, hamburger, lamb, pork, turkey
Avoid: None

Vegetables
Low oxalate: Acorn squash, alfalfa sprouts, white cabbage, cauliflower, cucumbers, green peas, iceberg lettuce, mung bean sprouts, red pepper, turnips, zucchini
Avoid: Beets, celery, eggplant, escarole, kale, leeks, parsley, green peppers, sweet potatoes, pumpkin, spinach, yellow squash, tomato sauce, watercress, yams

Desserts and Other Sweets
Low oxalate: Honey, jelly, jam, preserves, maple syrup, sugar, carob, gelatin
Avoid: Chocolate, fig newtons, fruitcake, marmalade, cocoa

Hormones and Vulvodynia: The New Treatment Link

Many researchers have long believed that hormones play a significant role in orchestrating vulvar pain. Although no one is certain what the exact link is, it's clear that for many women, vulvodynia is a cyclical occurrence, with pain increasing and decreasing in response to hormone fluctuations linked to the menstrual cycle.

In light of that fact, some experts have theorized that hormones, particularly estrogen, may have some ability to reduce vulvar pain, particularly when used topically, as a vaginal cream. Vulvar pain expert Dr. John H. Willems, head of obstetrics and gynecology at the Scripps Clinic and Research Foundation in La Jolla, California, believes that because estrogen works to remodel and recondition vaginal tissue, a hormone-based cream may also help "heal" damaged tissue, particularly in women whose vulvar pain began in response to vaginal laser surgery or chemical treatment for genital warts.

Indeed, Willems's eight-year study of some 200 vulvodynia patients found that up to 77 percent who used topical estrogen cream twice daily experienced significant pain relief. Although the healing

AN EXPERT'S OPINION ON . . .

Panty Liners and Vulvar Pain

Q: I've been diagnosed with vulvar vestibulitis, and I've heard that this can come from wearing panty liners too often. Is this true ?

A: While it's not likely that panty liners caused your problem initially, according to Milwaukee, Wisconsin gynecologist Dr. Jessica Thomason, they can definitely be a contributing factor to your pain. Reporting in *Ob.Gyn. News,* Thomason reveals that over a recent two-year period, an astounding 20 percent of her vulvar vestibulitis patients whose pain did not respond to traditional medication did indeed use panty liners daily or almost daily. More than 90 percent used pads or panty liners as their major feminine hygiene product.

Because the links between this mechanical barrier form of protection and the development of vulvar pain have not been scientifically explored, there are no concrete reasons as to why the connection exists. One possible theory has to do with the physical rubbing of the pad against nerve endings; another theory holds that chemicals in the pad itself (see Chapter 9) may cause some type of irritation. However, regardless of the reason, according to Dr. Thomason, if you have vulvar pain, you should consider minimizing the use of these products.

process was slow—improvement was generally not seen for at least six weeks—within six months most of the patients found relief.

If you're concerned that estrogen cream might have some of the same hormonal backlash as the oral version, particularly an increased risk of uterine and possibly breast cancer, Willems believes there is no cause for concern. Since only a minuscule amount of the hormone is absorbed into the body, he says, natural estrogen levels are not disturbed. Indeed, studies show that patients' blood levels checked both before and during estrogen cream therapy, showed no increase, and there were no outward signs of estrogen overload.

There are however, a few caveats associated with this treatment. Once started, it must be used on an ongoing basis; discontinuing use will cause a relapse, and all original symptoms will return. On the positive side, however, you can develop a maintenance program, gradually reducing the dosage until far less is needed to maintain relief. Additionally, as the healing process progresses, many women develop an intense vulvar itch. While your first instinct may be to treat it as a yeast infection and reach for an over-the-counter product, Willems says to resist: neither these treatments nor steroid creams will help. Instead, he says, try to cope with the itch, knowing it's only temporary and that it's a sign of healing.

According to the Vulvar Pain Foundation, the course of estrogen treatment may be a bumpy ride, with both flare-ups and setbacks, particularly during times of stress or prior to the onset of each menstrual cycle. The good news, however, is that eventually you will have more pain-free days than painful ones, and your symptoms will eventually subside.

Cough Medicine and Vulvar Pain: The Ingredient That Could Help

The ingredient is guaifenesin, commonly found in cough medicines called antitussants, products used to help dissolve and thin mucus. So what's the connection to vulvar pain?

According to Dr. R. Paul St. Amand, endocrinologist and assistant clinical professor at the University of California Harbor, UCLA,

BIRTH CONTROL PILLS AND VULVAR PAIN

Q: Can birth control pills increase vulvar pain? I started experiencing more intense burning and raw irritation about two months after I started taking the Pill. Is this a coincidence—or something more?

A: Since hormones are thought to play a role in vulvar pain, and birth control pills are essentially a hormone-based treatment, they may influence vulvar pain. Indeed, reports have indicated that the majority of women say that vulvodynia does worsen with the use of some birth control pills. However, you should also be aware that sometimes hormones in the Pill can affect the vaginal environment, which in turn increases the risk of several forms of vaginitis, all of which can cause the burning vulvar symptoms you describe. Since that is the case, make certain to get a complete pelvic exam, including tests for yeast infections and BV (see Chapters 2 and 3) before deciding whether to discontinue Pill use.

studies show that when taken regularly guaifenesin helps reverse symptoms of fibromyalgia, a muscle and joint pain syndrome that has been linked with vulvodynia. Although he freely admits his research is limited, Amand theorizes it works by keeping cells from retaining abnormally high levels of phosphate and oxalate—not coincidentally, the same chemicals that Solomons and other researchers have found to be excessive in women with some forms of vulvar pain.

Although dosages of guaifenesin can vary greatly, from as little as 300 mg daily to a whopping 3,600 mg a day, it produces no significant side effects.

Like the estrogen cream, however, once therapy begins, it must be continued indefinitely, or symptoms do return. Additionally, the treatment can't be used in conjunction with any products containing salicylic acid, be they oral or topical. This includes aspirin, as well as many herbs, particularly products containing aloe vera. The reason, says Amand, is that the acid blocks the effects of guaifenesin, so treatment will be worthless. Other products to avoid, he says, include Listerine, castor oil, and Ben Gay.

Also be aware that guaifenesin can cause hypoglycemia (low blood sugar), so be certain to check with your doctor if you experience excessive hunger, dizziness, fainting, panic attacks, or excessive sweating, particularly before mealtime.

The High-Tech Way Of Eliminating Vulvar Pain

Among the more high-tech ways of dealing with vulvar pain is the use of biofeedback, a computerized method of analyzing muscle tension and then using that information to retrain the muscles to exist in a more relaxed state.

How can this help vulvar pain?

According to studies conducted by Dr. Howard Glazer, a New York city neurophysiologist and clinical professor of obstetrics and gynecology at Cornell University Medical College/New York Presbyterian Hospital, some women respond to chronic vulvar pain by tensing pelvic muscles. This, in turn, causes chronic spasms that ultimately can make the vulva feel worse. As the pain increases, the muscles continue to spasm even more, so that eventually you end up with what seems like an unbreakable cycle of pain. Indeed, Glazer reported that in some patients muscle tension was so intense it precluded any other vulvar pain treatment from having an effective result.

The answer, he says, is to break the cycle of pain. His method is a carefully supervised and highly individualized program of biofeedback.

During this treatment your doctor inserts a tiny electronic sensor into your vagina. Thin lead wires from the sensor are attached to a biofeedback instrument designed to measure muscle contractions. Basing its responses on individualized physiological feedback, the instrument directs you when to squeeze vaginal muscles, and when

AN EXPERT'S OPINION ON . . .

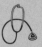

Vulvar Pain and Antidepressants

Q: A friend was just given antidepressant medication for her vulvar pain. Does this mean her doctor thinks it's all in her head?

A: Definitely not. According to experts from the University of Michigan Medical Center for Vulvar Diseases, one of the newer, and very effective, treatments for vulvar pain involves low doses of common tricyclic antidepressant medications amitriptyline (Elavil), desipramine (Norpramin), and nortriptyline (Pamelor). It is thought to work, say the experts, by inhibiting certain pain fibers that supply sensation to the vulva. This, in turn, can prevent the transmission of pain signals to the brain. Treatment generally must be used for three to six weeks before results are seen.

Doctors are also using small doses of anticonvulsant medications for a variety of chronic pain conditions, with some reports that these drugs may also work for vulvodynia.

In addition, speaking before the International Society for the Study of Vulvovaginal Disease World Congress, Milwaukee, Wisconsin gynecologist Dr. Jessica Thomason reported that her patients have also had favorable responses to still another type of antidepressant, medications known as SSRIs—selective serotonin reuptake inhibitors. The medications she found successful include sertraline (Zoloft) and paroxetine (Paxil), both of which helped vulvar pain, while minimizing side effects such as fatigue and constipation.

Doctors at New York Hospital–Cornell Medical Center found that antihistamines—the kind used to block an allergic reaction—helped women with vulvar pain. In their study of 220 women, 48.1 percent who tried these medications found pain relief. In addition, 77.0 percent of the women who tried injections of interferon, a type of immune stimulant drug, also found relief.

to release. The sensor, meanwhile, provides information about the strength of each contraction, as well as the amount of tension in the muscle when it is relaxed. With this information, you can learn to isolate pelvic floor muscles and then use various exercises to strengthen and tone them. Eventually, the painful muscle spasms are reduced or even completely disappear.

Additionally, pelvic muscles can become so stabilized that, even if the tension recurs, the pain does not.

Glazer's study of the method, published in the *Journal of Reproductive Medicine* in 1995, revealed that when properly supervised, these treatments were able to reduce pain in 80 percent of patients and eliminate it completely for nearly 50 percent of them. While improvement is not immediate—it takes about eight weeks of daily sessions to see results—after twelve weeks study participants found that pain was significantly diminished. After twenty-four weeks, most experienced a dramatic reduction in pain, and for some, it was completely gone.

AN EXPERT'S OPINION ON . . .

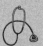

The Treatments to Avoid

According to the Vulvar Pain Foundation, there are a number of practitioners promoting treatments for vulvar pain that are not helpful, and in many instances may increase your pain. They say to be wary about accepting any of the following treatments:

- Alcohol injections
- Laser and incisional surgery
- Nerve blocks and neurectomies
- Podophyllin, fluorouracil (5-FU, Efudex) trichloroacetic acid (TCA)
- Most medicated creams, especially those that are cortisone based

Although the technology is still in its infancy, currently it is one of only a few noninvasive, nondrug treatments that has been scientifically demonstrated to effectively reduce vulvar pain.

Using high-tech electronics in a slightly different way, Dr. Mario Sideri, president of the International Society for the Study of Vulvovaginal Disease, treats patients with electric currents designed to passively relax pelvic muscles. The treatment, called functional antalgic electric stimulation, uses an electronic vaginal probe to relax pelvic muscles. Developed by Dr. Sideri at the European Institute of Oncology in Milan, Italy, it is usually administered for between nine and twenty-five minutes, three times a week, for a cycle consisting of twelve weeks. Sometimes up to three consecutive cycles are needed. However, according to studies conducted by Sideri, a seventeen-month follow-up treatment of fifty patients suffering with vulvar vestibulitis for twenty-four months or longer found that up to 90 percent experienced significant relief.

Self-Help for Easing Vulvar Pain

While medical treatment is the only way to cure your vulvar pain permanently, experts say there are a number of measures you can take to reduce your discomfort, particularly while you are receiving treatment. According to the Vulvar Pain Society, here are some things you can try:

- Take lukewarm baths several times daily. To further ease pain, add ½ cup of instant oatmeal, baking soda, or Aveeno to the water.
- Rinse your vulva after urination. If you do not have access to a bidet, invest in a plastic squirt bottle—but be certain to wash it and dry it thoroughly at least once a day.
- Rinse all your underwear at least twice in clean water. If you use a washing machine, run at least one cycle with clear water and no soap. This will help remove potentially irritating excess soap residues from fabric.
- Apply compresses of oatmeal, Aveeno, or wet tea bags for 5 to 10 minutes several times daily.

- Soothe your vulva with vitamin E oil several times daily or after urination.
- Use only 100 percent cotton menstrual pads; avoid tampons.
- Wear 100 percent cotton underwear; avoid panty hose.
- Avoid swimming in chlorinated water; avoid hot tubs.
- Avoid inhaling mold, mildew, and formaldehyde (found in carpets, pressed wood furniture, and nail polish).

When Sex Hurts and You Don't Know Why: What to Do

For an overwhelming majority of women, painful sex, particularly intercourse, is traced to vulvodynia—or sometimes a vaginal or urinary tract infection. When pain is felt deep within the vagina, as opposed to pain on entry, problems may be related to a pelvic condition, including endometriosis, pelvic inflammatory disease, adhesions, an ovarian cyst or tumor, or even a tear in the ligaments that support the uterus.

For a few women, pain can also occur with deep thrusting—when the penis hits the cervix and stimulates certain nerve endings—a problem that is often remedied by simply changing positions. And for some, an allergic response to a specific type of condom, a spermicide, or even an intimate care product such as a deodorant spray or a bath gel can all be linked to painful sex.

For some women, however, pain during intercourse is the result of a medical condition known as *dyspareunia*. In simplest terms, this is a lack of lubrication that makes friction between the penis and the vagina so painful that intercourse becomes difficult or impossible. Among the most common causes is inadequate stimulation prior to sex. More specifically, if your partner attempts intercourse before your body is physically ready, the result can be pain upon entry. If you don't feel as excited as you know you could be prior to intercourse, talk to your partner about what you can do together to extend foreplay. If this is not possible (some men simply get too excited, too fast), experts say you can try starting on your own, using masturbation to begin the stimulation and lubrication process. If problems

> ## DON'T USE THIS LUBRICANT— EVER!
>
> While petroleum jelly may temporarily ease painful sex, experts caution against using it for this purpose. The reason: this oil-based product does not dissolve in the vagina, so it might increase the growth of bacteria that ultimately lead to a vulvar infection.

continue even after stimulation is adequate, vulvar pain may be the result of a disorder in either the desire or excitement phase of sex—or more commonly, anxiety about upcoming sexual performance. In either case, talk to your doctor about treatment options such as hormone therapy, including estrogen creams.

You should also note that there is a natural reduction in lubrication that occurs during certain times of a woman's life, including during or right after menstruation, while breastfeeding, soon after childbirth, or in the years just prior to or right after menopause. When this is the case, often a simple lubricant, such as K-Y Jelly, Replens, or Astroglide, can provide all the lubrication you need. These products can also help when pain is the result of a lack of sexual stimulation by your partner.

Also helpful are lubricated tampons that you insert three times a week, for a continuous flow of soothing liquid. Although a bit costly, they are convenient, and there is some evidence that the constant lubrication may help reduce the risk of certain forms of vaginitis.

The Vaginal Muscle That Stops Sex

If, even after adequate lubrication, sex continues to be painful, and particularly if you cannot bear entry at all, you may be one of a small group of women affected by a muscle-related problem known as *vaginismus*. This occurs when muscles in the outer portion of your vagina contract to such a degree that penetration is extremely difficult. In essence, you tighten your vagina to such an extent that your partner's penis can't get through. Indeed, for some women, this same

TALKING POINT

If you have problems discussing painful sex with your doctor, you might try bringing up the subject in a slightly different way. Many women report that they start the conversation by asking their doctor what they might do to help increase their sexual responsiveness to their partner. Your doctor will likely take the cue and open the discussion for you.

problem occurs when they visit the gynecologist, often making it difficult or impossible to receive a pelvic exam.

Usually vaginismus is the result of previous sexual trauma or a current fear related to sexual activity, such as a dread of contracting HIV or even getting pregnant. Eventually the continual closing down of the vagina becomes an automatic response that occurs every time penetration is attempted.

If you believe this is the case for you, bring it to your doctor's attention. Often the treatment is a series of desensitization exercises you can do at home. Here, you will use your own fingers to gradually retrain your vaginal muscles to accept penetration. You will then move on to dilators of various sizes to help teach your muscles how to relax. In time, you will be encouraged to try intercourse again, in the female-superior position (woman on top), using your partner's erect penis as you would a dilator. Be certain, however, that both his penis and your vagina are liberally coated with lubricant.

A Final Word

If you are experiencing painful sex, be certain that you receive not only a complete pelvic exam but also blood tests, a Pap smear, a colposcopy (examination of the vagina under a microscope), and a pelvic ultrasound. If your pain is deep within your pelvis, you should also consider a laparoscopy, a minimally invasive surgery that allows your doctor a firsthand look inside your pelvic cavity. Indeed, the importance of this full exam cannot be emphasized enough, particularly to ensure you receive the best and quickest solution to your problem.

Certainly, if any obvious cause for your pain is found, such as an infection, treatment should be rendered immediately. Often this is all you will need to begin enjoying sex once again. If not, you can at least be certain that whatever other treatments you try, success is more likely when underlying medical problems are under control.

Also keep in mind that even with all the diagnostic and treatment advances available today, not all doctors are equally versed in the diagnosis and treatment of vulvar pain or painful sex. If you do suffer from the symptoms and problems described in this chapter and your doctor has not offered you any substantial relief, make certain to get a second, and if need be, a third opinion.

Most important, know that you do not have to suffer in silence— and you do not have to suffer alone. Your pain can be reduced and in many instances even eliminated with the right care.

CHAPTER SIX

Burning Desire

Overcoming Urinary Tract Infections

They can develop without warning, seemingly without rhyme or reason. Or they can follow a definite pattern, mimicking a menstrual cycle, occurring after sex, or for some women, every time they get a gynecological exam.

The problem is UTIs—short for urinary tract infections, a problem affecting upwards of 26 million women every year, many between the ages of eighteen and thirty-five. And while men can develop these infections as well, women, it seems, are up to twenty-five times more likely to be affected. One reason, say experts, has to do with our basic anatomy. A woman's body makes it far easier for bacteria to invade the urinary tract and cause problems.

Indeed, the female urethra—the tube that carries urine out of the body—is only a scant 1 inch long, making it relatively easy for any bacteria in the V zone to find their way to the urinary tract. But where does that bacteria come from to begin with? You may be surprised to learn that most of the time it's right from your own body. Indeed, while there are a number of micro-organisms capable of causing a UTI (including enterobacteria, pseudomonas, and staphylococcus), most infections are the result of the *Escherichia coli* bacteria, found naturally in the digestive tract, in stool, around the anus, and on the skin between the anus and the vagina. When, due to any number of situations (and we'll get specific in a minute) *E. coli* or any other bacteria make their way inside the urethra, they adhere to the cell wall and begin to multiply. In not too long a time, they begin to travel through the short tubing to the bladder, where they attach to the lining and cause an irritation (see illustration). This causes the bladder to begin contracting as if trying to push the unwanted bacteria from its cell walls. It is actually these contractions that trigger the urgent need to urinate that often accompanies a UTI. The same bacteria also irritate the urethra, so much so that when they come in contact with the normal acid found in urine, an intense burning sensation (called dysuria) can occur.

Regardless of the type of bacteria causing your UTI, your infection will normally fall into one of three categories; according to the National Bladder Foundation (NBF), they are:

Urethritis—an infection of the urethra usually causing pain and burning during urination.

Cystitis—an infection in the bladder that in addition to pain and burning, also causes frequent urination and the urgent need to urinate with little passage of actual urine. Often urethritis and cystitis occur together.

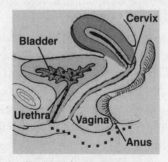

HOW BACTERIA TRAVEL

Most UTIs occur when bacteria that normally reside in the digestive tract and stool make their way to the area of skin between the anus and vagina, where they can quickly and easily migrate into the urethra, a tube just one inch long leading directly to the bladder. Once there, they attach to the bladder wall and begin to grow, thus causing a urinary tract infection to develop.

Pyelonephritis—a kidney infection that is less common than the two other forms of UTIs but can be more serious. In addition to symptoms mentioned above, you may also experience fever, chills, backache, bloody or cloudy urine, nausea, and vomiting.

In addition, the NBF suggests, many women who experience any type of UTI often feel "bad all over"—tired, shaky, washed out, and generally achy. There can also be pain in and around the pubic bone area, even when not urinating, and occasionally leaking urine, which may have a slightly foul odor.

Sex and UTIs: What You Need to Know

Although there are some women for whom UTIs appear to just happen, often there are one or more contributing factors increasing the risk. This is particularly the case for women with repeated infections, occurring more than once or twice a year. Among the most common of those factors is sexual intercourse.

Because vaginal walls are so close to the urethra, it gets vigorously rubbed during sex. This causes swelling and inflammation, which then makes it easier for bacteria to take hold. More important, the rubbing action also causes any bacteria normally found in the vagina or on the skin anywhere within the V zone to be pushed directly into the urethra, where they can take hold, begin to multiply, and then quickly ascend into the bladder.

All of these possibilities increase with the frequency with which you have intercourse, with the most problems occurring with repeated acts that occur over a relatively short period of time (for example, three times a day for three or more days). Heavy penile thrusting can also increase risks, as can anal intercourse followed by vaginal penetration. Indeed, experts suggest that if you do engage in anal sex, be certain that your partner thoroughly washes his penis before inserting it into your vagina, even if he uses a condom for both sex acts. Remember that the condom can protect your V zone only from what is on or in his penis. Often *E. coli* bacteria that linger in and around the anus attach to his entire "P" zone, so any area of his genitalia can easily transmit those bacteria to your urethra.

AN EXPERT'S OPINION ON . . .

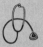

Sex, Viagra, and UTIs

Q: Three days into what I thought was going to be a superromantic Hawaiian vacation, I developed the worst UTI I've ever had. It hurt so bad we had to stop having sex for the rest of the trip. But when I got home, my test was negative for bacteria. My doctor said not to worry and then asked what I thought was a totally weird question—if my husband was using Viagra. And he was! What's the connection here?

A: According to reports in a 1998 *New England Journal of Medicine*, a group of Georgia physicians noticed a rise in female patients with UTIs in a strange pattern that coincided with the increase in the number of their male patients who were taking Viagra. After a little investigation, Dr. Henry Patton says, "Out of 100 men who got Viagra, 15 of their wives came to us with cystitis." Since publishing their findings in the *Journal,* the Georgia doctors say they have heard from physicians around the nation who report similar findings.

As to whether Viagra has some residual ejaculatory-related chemical effect on a woman, the answer is that it is highly unlikely. What is more likely to be true, say experts, is that the increase in sexual activity encouraged by the Viagra is the real culprit here. In a condition known as "honeymoon cystitis," the urethra, which is located very close to the vagina, becomes swollen and irritated as the result of intercourse, including frequent, forceful penetration. When the acid in urine (or sometimes irritants found in spermicides or lubricants) comes in contact with the inflamed tissue, the burning pain you normally associate with a UTI is felt.

(continued on next page)

Although it's possible for some bacteria to make their way into the urethra during repeated acts of intercourse, when honeymoon cystitis is the issue, often the culture is negative for any offending organisms.

To avoid problems in the future, make certain your vagina is adequately lubricated before each act of intercourse (if necessary, use a nonirritating substance such as Astroglide to help), and try to empty your bladder *before* intercourse, to relieve any extra pressure. Most important, if you begin to feel a sense of irritation, hide your honey's Viagra and give your V zone a rest! Avoiding intercourse for as little as twelve hours can help tissue repair itself.

Birth Control and UTIs: The New Links

Can your choice of birth control increase your risk of a UTI? Experts say that it can (see illustration). Indeed, according to the NBF, studies show that women who use the diaphragm method of preventing pregnancy are two to three times more prone to UTIs than those who use other forms, and doctors have provided a variety of theories as to why. In some instances, experts say it is not so much the device but the size that makes the difference, with larger diaphragms putting too much pressure on the urethra, which in turn causes an irritation that ultimately allows bacteria to take hold. In addition, a large diaphragm may constrict urine flow by putting pressure on the bladder—and that in turn may increase risk of infection.

In either case, the solution lies in getting the smallest possible size diaphragm and being certain to have it refitted if you lose a significant amount of weight. Additionally, some anecdotal reports indicate that diaphragms with soft rather than firm outside rims may cause less pressure, and consequently may not increase your risk of UTIs quite as much.

There are also some experts who believe that the real link to UTIs may not be the diaphragm itself but rather the products used along with it, such as spermicides and jellies. At least three important stud-

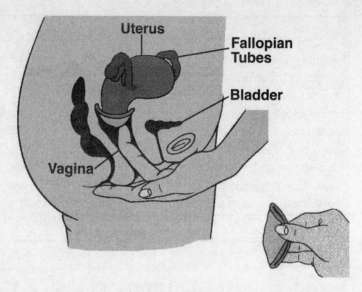

BIRTH CONTROL AND UTIS

If you use the diaphragm method of birth control, make certain that it fits snugly against your cervix, and get the smallest size possible. These precautions will help reduce the restriction of urine flow that sometimes occurs when the diaphragm is improperly fitted, particularly if it is too large. Additionally, units with a soft rather than a hard rim (see insert at lower right) may further help reduce the risk of related urinary tract infections.

Courtesy of Lippincott, Williams & Wilkins, Medi-Clip

ies—one conducted at Toronto General Hospital, and two at the University of Washington's Harborview Medical Center in Seattle—have shown that at least one intimate product ingredient, the spermicide nonoxynol-9, increased the risk of both bladder and yeast infections in women. Even when used without a diaphragm, products containing nonoxynol-9 carried the same risk of infection.

Although doctors aren't certain what that link is, some believe it may be that vaginal irritation occurs when delicate tissue comes in contact with the spermicide. This may make it easier for bacteria to proliferate and then readily ascend to the urethra and into the bladder.

Another theory cites the negative effects that nonoxynol-9 appears

MEN, SEX, AND UTIs

Q: Do men get UTIs, and is it possible for a woman to catch one from a man during sex?

A: Yes, men do get UTIs, but not nearly as often as women do. The main reason is the longer male urethral pathway, which means bacteria must travel a lot farther in order to reach a man's bladder. When men do get a UTI, it's usually the result of an obstruction in the urinary tract, such as a kidney stone or an enlarged prostate.

As to "catching" his UTI during sex, it's not likely, mostly because the infection is in his bladder. Presumably he won't urinate during intercourse, so the bacteria won't get into your body.

That said, it is possible that bacteria from his infection may be lurking in his P zone, in which case intimate contact may put you in touch with the same germs. If they make it from your vagina into your urethra, you could end up with a UTI.

to have on the "good" bacteria found in a woman's V zone. Specifically, studies show it may kill off lactobacillus, which helps women avoid intimate infections by keeping the *E. coli* bacteria in check. Indeed, when levels of lactobacillus go down, the proliferation of *E. coli* goes up, and some may find their way to the urethra. Supporting this line of thinking, experts at the National Institute of Diabetes and Digestive and Kidney Diseases (NIDDK) report that when tested, women whose partners use a condom with spermicide are more likely to have *E. coli* bacteria in their vagina.

Diagnosis and Treatment: How Your Doctor Can Help

Although the symptoms of a UTI are hard to miss, it's important that you at least consult with your doctor each time problems arise. First,

UTIs AND PELVIC EXAMS

Q: It seems that almost every time I have my annual pelvic exam, I end up with a UTI. I'm beginning to wonder if I'm not picking up this infection in my doctor's office. Is it possible?

A: While you're not likely to "catch" a UTI, as you would a cold or flu, it's possible that your pelvic exam may be playing a role. Sometimes bacteria normally residing outside your vagina may be pushed inside, near the urethra, during your pelvic exam, particularly if your doctor uses any type of instruments, such as an ultrasound vaginal probe.

To help avoid problems, try drinking a glass of water right before your exam, then urinating right afterward. This will help flush the bacteria from your urethra before they can hang around long enough to cause problems. Also, talk to your doctor about your suspicions. He or she may be able to take a few extra precautions during the exam itself to prevent further problems.

you will likely need a prescription antibiotic in order for the infection to clear. While some milder UTIs can sometimes go away on their own, more often than not, experts say that when left untreated, they can evolve into more serious infections that are infinitely more difficult to cure.

This brings us to the second reason not to avoid medical care: occasionally a UTI will progress to a much more serious kidney infection, sometimes with little or no warning. Studies show that up to 30 percent of women whose symptoms might otherwise indicate a simple UTI are really suffering from what is medically known as a silent kidney infection—a serious, even life-threatening condition that is a lot worse than it feels at the moment.

The best way to avoid any unnecessary problems, as well as getting your UTI under swift control, is to call your doctor as soon as symptoms appear. What will he or she do?

AN EXPERT'S OPINION ON . . .

Menstrual Cycles, Stress, and UTIs

Q: I've begun to notice that my UTIs always occur right around the time of my monthly cycle, sometimes three or four times a year. Could there be any connection?

A: According to reports in the journal *Women's Urological Health,* the answer is likely yes, with the underlying cause being the reproductive hormone estrogen.

Studies show that when estrogen levels decline, as they do right after the start of each menstrual cycle, you also experience a decline in levels of the "good" lactobacillus bacteria, which helps keep *E. coli* in check. With less lactobacillus around to protect your V zone, it's far easier for the *E. coli* lurking in the vicinity to jump in and take hold—and begin growing out of control. If in the process they work their way into your urethra, it's just a short skip to the bladder, where the infection can begin. Before you know it, a UTI has developed.

In addition, if you suffer from PMS, the stress associated with these symptoms may also increase your odds of menstrual-related urinary infections. Experts say that often a UTI will develop following a stress-filled event, or sometimes in anticipation of one. So if your periods are exceptionally difficult for you due to either PMS or menstrual pain, doing what you can to reduce stress levels during each cycle may help you avoid a UTI.

You should also note that any condition or situation that suppresses or even taxes your immune system, such as diabetes or cancer, may also increase your risk of a UTI, either during your menstrual cycle or at any other time.

First, you will be asked to give what is called a "clean-catch" sample of your urine. To accomplish this, you will wash your genitals with warm water (this will help remove any V zone bacteria that might otherwise end up in your urine sample), then urinate into a sterile container. Your sample is then analyzed under a microscope for the presence of bacteria and pus.

Your doctor may also offer you a urine culture. Here, any bacteria found in your urine are grown in a lab to help identify the exact germ causing your infection. Although getting the results takes about two days, it can help zero in on the specific medication you need to eradicate your UTI quickly and effectively.

The most common and the most effective treatment is oral antibiotic—and there is a variety of drugs from which to choose. While in the past, treatment often required seven to fourteen days of therapy to cure an infection, newer, stronger, more effective drugs have significantly decreased the time it takes to get well.

Today most often doctors prescribe just a three-day regimen—and for some women, a single-dose regimen is all that's needed to eradicate the bacterium. According to the NIDDK, among the most commonly used medications for UTIs are these:

- Trimethoprim (Trimpex)
- Trimethoprim/sulfamethoxazole (Bactrim, Septra, Cotrim)
- Amoxicillin (Amoxil, Trimox, Wymox)
- Nitrofurantoin (Macrodantin, Furadantin, Macrobid)
- Fosfomycin tromethamine (Monurol)
- Sulfonamides
- Penicillin
- Quinolones, which are particularly important in the treatment of drug-resistant strains of *E. coli*.

Usually the exact drug and the specific dosage are determined by both the type of bacteria found in your urine culture and your personal health history. One-dose regimens, for example, should always be avoided if you have delayed treatment of your symptoms, if you have any signs of kidney infection, if you are diabetic, or if you are pregnant.

Regardless of which treatment your doctor prescribes, once you begin, you can expect relief to come fairly quickly. In most instances a few doses will likely relieve your urgent need to urinate and any pain in your bladder. Within two or three more days, the rest of your symptoms, including the burning urination, should quit.

Remember, however, always to take your complete prescription, even if it seems as if the problem is gone within a few doses. Stopping your medication before your UTI is effectively cleared could increase your risk of developing a more serious kidney infection.

If your UTI does affect your kidney, the Infectious Disease Society of America suggests you may still require up to fourteen days of antibiotic treatment. In some instances an oral medication, alone or combined with an injection, may be needed. In rare instances you may be hospitalized, so that more potent intravenous drugs can be administered.

Pregnancy and UTIs

According to the NBF, up to 4 percent of pregnant women develop UTIs. Hormonal shifts, as well as the physiological changes that occur as the baby grows, can make it easier for bacteria to proliferate and quickly travel through the urinary tract. Moreover, UTIs that occur during pregnancy are often more severe than at other times, sometimes leading to a kidney infection. If not treated early on, this can threaten a mother's life, as well as increase the risk of premature labor. For this reason, the American College of Obstetrics and Gynecology suggests your first pregnancy exam should always include a urine culture for infection, and you should be tested at intervals throughout your pregnancy.

If you should develop the symptoms of a UTI, the NBF says to seek medical help immediately. While many antibiotics are not recommended for use during pregnancy, a few, including the drug cephalexin, are effective and safe. If your infection is particularly severe, you can expect your doctor to recommend that you continue taking low doses of antibiotic for several weeks after your UTI clears.

In addition, you should be aware that your risk of a UTI also in-

AN EXPERT'S OPINION ON . . .

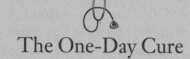

The One-Day Cure

Q: I've heard that a one-dose treatment is available for UTIs, yet my doctor says three to seven days is still the best. I'm wondering whether he's giving me more medicine than I need, and that concerns me.

A: Certainly it's always best to limit medication to only as much as you need, and no more. One reason is antibiotic resistance, a growing problem that limits the effect of common medications on certain bacteria, including those that cause a UTI. That said, by insisting that you take medication for the full seven days, your doctor may be erring on the side of caution, and there is some new research to show he is right.

According to analysis presented at the Thirty-ninth Annual Interscience Conference on Antimicrobial Agents and Chemotherapy in 1999, there appears to be no solid evidence that single-dose therapy is better than or even equal to longer therapy.

The latest recommendation is that at least three days of treatment with trimethoprim/sulfamethoxazole (Bactrim, Septra, Cotrim) is the best treatment for an uncomplicated UTI.

creases in the forty-eight hours following delivery. Because your body needs to get rid of a lot of excess fluid quickly following birth, your urine output increases, sometimes to as much as 4 cups at a time. Giving in to that frequent urge to urinate may help you avoid a UTI. At the same time, some women find it difficult to urinate after childbirth, thus allowing not only the excess fluid to build but also increasing the risk that bacteria can develop. When this is the case, your doctor may recommend a catheter (a thin, flexible tube) to remove the urine from your bladder. This will not only help reduce your risk of a UTI, but also make it possible to test your urine to ensure that an infection has not set in.

When More Testing Is Needed: What to Do

If your UTI was also accompanied by fever, if blood was found in your urine, or if you don't respond to antibiotic treatment, further

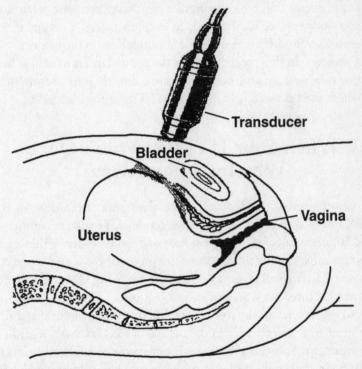

THE ABDOMINAL ULTRASOUND EXAM

If your UTI does not respond to treatment, and particularly if you are experiencing fever, pain, or blood in the urine, an ultrasound exam can help. Completely painless, and taking just minutes to perform, it involves the use of a wandlike transducer that your doctor will pass over the outside of your pelvis and kidneys to image any abnormalities that could be contributing to your infection.

Courtesy of Lippincott, Williams & Wilkins, Medi-Clip

testing may be needed to ensure against possible damage to your kidneys. When this is the case, one of these three tests can help:

- *Intravenous pyelogram (IVP).* Here, opaque dye is injected into a vein, so that an X ray can be taken of your bladder, kidneys, and ureter. This will help reveal the presence of any defects in structure, as well as any blockages due to tumors or even scar tissue from previous UTIs.
- *Ultrasound exam.* Similar to a vaginal ultrasound, in this instance your doctor will pass a wandlike structure over your pelvis and your kidneys (see illustration). In some instances, a vaginal sonogram can also help reveal certain abnormalities in the bladder.
- *Cystoscopy.* In this procedure your doctor will insert a narrow, hollow tube with an attached light source directly into your urethra, which then allows a field of vision as far up as the bladder.

When Your UTI Just Won't Quit: Why Infections Recur

For most women, UTIs occur more than once. According to the NBF, nearly 20 percent of those who get one UTI will get another— and 30 percent of *those* will get at least one more—often within eighteen months. If you fall into the latter group, there is an 80 percent chance that you will go on to experience recurring UTIs, sometimes as many as three per year, year in and year out.

No one is certain why this occurs, but one theory holds that a single strain of *E. coli* remains in the vaginal or fecal reservoir, regardless of treatment. So from almost the moment the medication is out of your body, that strain begins to multiply, and before long it makes its way to your urethra. But what makes the *E. coli* multiply in the first place?

According to Dr. Robert Moldwin, assistant professor of urology at Albert Einstein College of Medicine in New York City, problems may originate within the cells lining the bladder and even the vagina. In this instance, he says, the cells themselves may undergo some type of change that makes them "stickier," thus allowing bacteria that might otherwise be flushed from the body naturally to remain attached to the cell wall. Since both the vagina and the bladder are conducive environments for bacteria to grow, once attached, they begin to multiply, setting the wheels in motion for a UTI to develop.

Similarly, a recent NIH-funded study found that certain factors present in the blood of some women may predispose them to UTIs, mainly by allowing bacteria to attach more easily to the cells lining the vagina and urethra.

One problem that is often overlooked as a potential cause of recurring UTIs is an infection in the Skene gland. These tiny glands lo-

AN EXPERT'S OPINION ON . . .

Risk Factors for UTIs

Data presented by Dr. Walter Stamm at the Thirty-ninth Interscience Conference on Antimicrobial Agents and Chemotherapy in September 1999 suggests that risk factors for recurring UTIs in women now include the following:

- Spermicide use
- Four sexual encounters per month or more
- New sex partner in the past year
- Maternal history of UTI
- First UTI before age fifteen

What isn't likely to cause a recurring UTI? According to Stamm:

- Douching
- Voiding habits before or after intercourse
- BV or STDs
- Bathroom wiping patterns
- Tub bathing
- Types of underwear
- Infected sex partners

cated at the end of the urethral opening right near the entry to the vagina normally secrete mucus to help keep the entire area lubricated. Occasionally, however, they can become clogged, causing pus to build and fill the inner cavity. This creates a reservoir of bacteria that continually infect the urethra. Most of the time, an antibiotic will clear the infection, and the UTIs will stop. In some instances, however, when the infections continue to recur, the glands must be removed before the UTIs will stop.

Solutions:
The Treatments That Can Help

If you are plagued with recurring UTIs, there are a few specific treatment regimens you may want to explore. Should you experience three or more UTIs within twelve months, you should consider talking to your doctor about one of the following treatment plans.

Option #1: Continuous Low-Dose Antibiotic Therapy

In this instance you will take small daily doses of one of two antibiotics—sometimes the trimethoprim/sulfamethoxazole combination regimen, or more recently recommended, nitrofurantoin. In National Institutes of Health research conducted by the University of Washington in Seattle, doctors found that not only is low-dose nitrofurantoin effective, but long-term daily usage poses no serious side effects.

Option #2: Single-Dose Antibiotic Therapy After Sex

The theory here is that taking a one-dose pill of antibiotic directly after intercourse will help stamp out any bacteria that made their way into your urethra, before they have a chance to multiply and ascend to your bladder. According to some experts, the antibiotic Macrodantin is particularly effective in this therapy, since it remains mostly in the bladder.

Option #3: Short-Term Antibiotic Therapy as Symptoms Begin

Here you will be asked to pay special attention to your body. At the first sign that a UTI may be approaching, you will take antibiotics for up to two days. What can also help: Urine dipsticks, available at the drugstore without a prescription. They help diagnose an impending infection by detecting nitrite, a chemical that forms in the urine when bacteria are present. Performing the test on a regular basis can help catch up to 90 percent of infections at their earliest stages, often before symptoms appear. Taking medication right away will keep the infection from escalating.

Self-Start Therapy: The Latest News

The newest treatment for recurring UTIs involves a twist on the short-term antibiotic option. Called *self-start therapy,* according to experts at the Northwestern University Medical School in Chicago, where studies took place, patients were given a home diagnostic kit containing a urine culture test and six tablets of norfloxacin, 400 mg each. Using the self-generated urine culture, they were encouraged to test their own urine frequently, particularly after sex or with the first hint of symptoms.

If at any time the culture tested positive for the presence of bacteria, the women were instructed to begin the medication regimen and visit their doctor within five to nine days for follow-up testing and any necessary additional medication. Four to six weeks later, another follow-up visit was required.

According to the Northwestern studies, published in the *Journal of Urology* in 1999, not only was it a safe and effective way of controlling recurring UTIs, it also turned out to be an exceedingly economical form of care.

AN EXPERT'S OPINION ON . . .

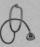

Chocolate Bars and UTIs

Q: Can eating too much sugar cause a UTI? I'm embarrassed to tell my doctor that every time I binge out on chocolate, I end up with a urinary infection. Will he think I'm nuts?

A: While there is no evidence that sweets can bring on a UTI in *normal* folks, your bingeing could indicate a blood sugar problem, which *is* connected to an increased risk of urinary tract infections.

According to a 1995 study in the *Journal of Women's Health,* diabetics are twice as likely to develop UTIs as are women with normal sugar levels. Although no one is certain why, many believe that higher-than-normal sugar levels change the vaginal environment, making it far easier for V zone bacteria to grow out of control. When they do, they can easily ascend into the urethra and then the bladder, causing recurring problems. And since diabetes can injure the kidneys, these infections can be doubly worrisome.

To be certain this isn't your problem, confide your symptoms to your doctor and ask for a six-hour glucose tolerance test. If your chocolate binges are tied to a blood sugar problem, your UTIs may be the result of too many candy bars.

Is It Really a UTI? How to Tell

Because there are a number of conditions and infections that can be confused with a UTI, including vaginitis and some sexually transmitted diseases, a diagnosis isn't always easy. Moreover, in some women symptoms prevail but no infection of any kind can be found in the urine—making it even harder to track down the problem.

That's why, sometimes, diagnosis becomes a matter of elimination, with a round of testing performed to rule out such problems as vaginitis, STDs, and allergies. A cystoscope exam, which looks inside the bladder, can also help eliminate the possibility that a structural problem may be the source of symptoms.

If all of these tests produce negative results, meaning no infection is found, your doctor may suggest simple treatments designed to offer some comfort and relief, such as warm sitz baths or medications that reduce bladder pain, including Pyridium (which can turn urine bright red), or methenamine (Prosed, Urised), which can turn urine bright blue. You can also ask your druggist about the over-the-counter medication phenazopyridine hydrochloride—but only if all tests show negative results.

If problems persist in spite of negative test results, you may be suffering from one of the following conditions :

Chronic urinary tract irritability. This is the result of a dysfunctional voiding reflex, a problem characterized by the urgent need to urinate even when the bladder isn't full. And because it isn't, the necessary contractions needed to push urine out do not occur.

Chronically tight pelvic muscles. In this instance, the entire hammock of muscle holding your lower urinary tract in place can become so tense that it creates pressure on the bladder, which in turn increases the risk of symptoms.

Irritable bladder. If you suffered with urinary tract problems in childhood, you may simply end up with a bladder that overreacts to stimulation as an adult. Similar problems can occur as the result of certain pelvic surgeries, a thyroid disorder, or some neurological diseases, as well as irritable bowel syndrome.

Fibroid tumors. Occasionally these benign uterine growths can press on the bladder, causing a variety of symptoms, including those associated with a UTI. Medication or surgery to remove the fibroid can help.

Interstitial cystitis (IC). Also known as "burning bladder," this somewhat mysterious ailment causes intense pain during urination as well as a constant urge to urinate and a bladder that becomes painful as soon as it begins to fill. According to the Interstitial Cystitis Foundation, there is no bacterial link to this disease. Instead, symptoms occur as a result of inflammation in the space between the lining of the bladder and the muscle wall. While IC often does begin as a UTI, the pain and other urinary problems continue long after the infection is cleared. Often treatment will require a urologist who specializes in IC.

Nine Ways to Avoid a UTI

Certainly the best way to prevent UTIs from recurring is to seek medical attention at the first sign of any symptoms. But is there anything

---

SYMPTOM-FREE UTIs

Q: I recently had a routine urine analysis as part of a physical for my new job. I was shocked to discover I had what the doctor called a raging UTI. I had no symptoms of any kind, and now I'm wondering if this doctor knew what he was talking about or if my test results were confused with someone else's.

A: Certainly it's possible that the lab did make a mistake, so it's probably a good idea to have a repeat test. However, you should also know that up to 5 percent of all sexually active women and up to 15 percent of all women over age sixty are affected by what is medically known as asymptomatic bacteriuria, or ASB, a urinary tract infection that is usually symptom free.

Certainly whether you have symptoms or not, any UTI diagnosed by your doctor should be treated with appropriate medications. This is particularly important during pregnancy, since any threat of kidney infection also increases the risk of premature labor and high blood pressure in the mother.

Mother Nature's Bounty
Cranberry Juice, Yogurt,
and Echinacea

For decades both women and their doctors have been musing over the health benefits of cranberry juice, particularly as a preventative for UTIs. While reports of the "cranberry cure" were almost legendary, they were in fact only anecdotal, with no real scientific proof to support the claims.

Now, however, that has changed, thanks to a new study conducted by Brigham and Women's Hospital and Harvard Medical School in Boston. They found that cranberry juice *does* appear to have protective properties and may help you avoid a UTI. The patient study, which involved 153 women, was randomly divided into two groups. One group drank 10 ounces of cranberry juice daily for six months, and the other drank a taste-alike drink with no cranberries. At the end of the six months, urine samples were taken from all the women. The result: While 28 percent of those drinking the noncranberry drink had pus and bacteria in their urine, only 15 percent in the cranberry juice group were similarly affected. Since bacteria increase the risk of a UTI, doctors say the juice appears to help reduce the risk of infection.

Although the study was sponsored by Ocean Spray, which processes and sells cranberry juice, the findings were nonetheless considered unbiased and true. There was, however, one surprising result. While doctors always believed that the effectiveness of cranberry juice came from its ability to make urine more acidic, thus keeping bacteria at bay, the new study showed this is not so. Instead, its protective quality is that of an antiadhesive, preventing *E. coli* bacteria from sticking to the bladder wall.

In addition, while it wasn't a part of this particular study, some naturopathic physicians now recommend adding a teaspoon of tincture of echinacea to your cranberry juice three times a day.

Working as an immune stimulant, it is thought to help increase the body's own germ-fighting powers, destroying bacteria before they can proliferate. If you try this, however, don't be surprised to experience a tingling, almost numbing feeling on your tongue for several minutes afterwards. It's normal and harmless.

It is important to note, however, that with or without echinacea, cranberry juice is highly acidic, so if you already have a UTI, it could make symptoms worse. To avoid problems, try diluting the juice with lots of water. Or you could just eat blueberries. Studies show they contain the same protective phytochemicals as cranberries, with a lot less acid.

Additionally, while scientific reports remain largely anecdotal in nature, many doctors now believe that eating a daily dose of yogurt containing live lactobacillus cultures may have some protective effects as well. The link, say experts, is that the acid in the yogurt works to discourage the growth of bacteria. Even less scientific—but some say more useful—is the practice of placing yogurt *directly in the vagina,* particularly near the opening of the urethra. Since yogurt does contain acid, don't try this if your V zone tissue is already inflamed. In addition, never use yogurt that contains sugar, since this will help increase the growth of bacteria. Also be certain to cleanse your genitals thoroughly after a V zone yogurt treatment.

Finally, Judyth Reichenberg-Ullman, N.D., M.S.W., suggests that herbal tinctures may also provide relief, especially when taken in small doses throughout the day. Her recommendations for bladder infections are: *Barosma betulina* (buchu), *Chimaphilla* (pipsissewa), *Berberis aquifolia* (Oregon grape), and *Uva ursi* (bearberry). Reichenberg-Ullman also recommends goldenseal, corn silk, and marshmallow root. Her top suggestion: "Drink, drink drink! Be certain to drink as much water as you possibly can during an acute bladder infection."

you can do to keep even an initial infection from occurring? Many experts say yes. There are, in fact, a number of preventative strategies you can and should take, particularly if you have had one or more UTIs in the past. According to experts at the University of Iowa Women's Health Center, Department of Obstetrics and Gynecology at the University of Iowa, here are some guidelines that can help:

- Drink eight to ten glasses of water daily. This will help increase your amount of urine output, which will allow you to flush your bladder and urethra more frequently—and that can help reduce your risk of infection.
- Pay close attention to personal hygiene. This includes making certain to wash your genitals with soap and warm water, particularly after sex, and remembering to change sanitary napkins or tampons at least several times a day during your menstrual cycle. In addition, for many years doctors also recommended that you always wipe yourself from front to back (and not the other way around) to avoid spreading *E. coli* bacteria found naturally near your anus, upward toward your urethra. Now, however, at least some doctors debate the importance of this action in the development of UTIs.
- Reduce your intake of spicy foods, as well as high-acid liquids such as coffee, caffeinated or carbonated beverages, and alcohol. These foods and beverages won't give you a UTI, but they can irritate your bladder, making an existing infection feel worse or even increasing inflammation, making it easier for bacteria to proliferate.
- Avoid nylon crotch panties, tight jeans, and panty hose. These items can hold in body heat, making it easier for bacteria to grow.
- Avoid perfumed toilet paper, bubble bath, bath oils, dusting powder, and scented soaps. These items won't cause a UTI, but they can increase inflammation and symptoms. The same can be said of some tampons and sanitary napkins, particularly those containing deodorants or scents (see Chapter 9).
- Don't hold in urine, and don't rush when you do urinate, making certain to empty your bladder completely. This can help flush out the bacteria before they have a chance to take hold and multiply.
- Cleanse genitals before sex and urinate as soon after intercourse as possible. Again, this will help flush bacteria from the bladder.

- Use a heating pad and frequent warm baths to help ease the pain of a UTI, and rinse your genitals with plain warm water after urinating to reduce the acid burn on the urethra.
- Don't smoke. It increases the risk of bladder cancer.

On the Horizon:
Treatments in the New Millennium

If a certain group of researchers is right, UTIs may one day cease to exist. The reason is a powerful new vaccine, one that has proven so successful in animal studies it is now being tested in humans. It works, say experts, by blocking a protein that *E. coli* needs to attach itself to the wall of the bladder. With this function disabled, any bacteria that find their way up the urethra will be flushed out during normal urination.

Until the day when UTIs are a thing of the past, you can help stave off serious infections with early detection, courtesy of a number of new home test kits headed for the market. At least one of those kits, appropriately called the UTI, is available now. It comes with six urine collection cups and a handful of test strips, which are placed in the urine specimen to confirm the presence of most bacteria linked to UTIs. The kit can also be used to monitor the effectiveness of treatment for recurring infections.

CHAPTER SEVEN

When Good Girls Get Bad Diseases

A Guide to Sexually Transmitted Infections

When you think of the word *sex,* what other terms come to mind? *Pleasure? Fun? Romance? Passion?*

You may even be thinking, "All of the above!"

In today's world, however, there are a few more words every woman must now also associate with sex—and they include *safety, caution,* and *infection.*

The reason is sexually transmitted diseases, or STDs. And while it was once believed that only "bad girls" need worry about these infections, today we know how wrong that kind of thinking is. Indeed, changes in our culture, including sexual experiences beginning at a younger age, combined with marrying older and divorcing more often, mean that all of us have more sex partners and more frequent encounters than ever before. And that, in turn, increases everyone's risk of contracting an STD.

Moreover, while we may be getting closer to living in an equal opportunity world, unfortunately, the same can't be said for sexually transmitted diseases. For the most part, STDs *are not* equal opportunity bugs. According to studies conducted by the U.S. Department of Health and Human Services, it is women, and not men, who bear the brunt of these diseases, in terms of both risks and complications.

Indeed, many STDs are far easier for a woman to acquire from a man than the other way around. Studies as far back as 1984 revealed

women are twice as likely as men to contract two of the most prevalent STDs, chlamydia and gonorrhea, *during a single sexual encounter.*
The newest studies show that women are twenty times more likely
than men to contract HIV. Why?

Part of the problem has to do with our anatomy. A woman's reproductive system is filled with so many dark, warm spaces that it's far
easier for infections to take hold and thrive in our body, than in a
man's body.

But that's not the whole reason. Sex, it seems, also increases our
risks—and not just in the transmission of these nasty bugs. Semen
has a neutralizing effect on the vagina, reducing the normally acidic,
protective environment to a buffered, alkaline zone that favors the
growth of bacteria. So every time your partner ejaculates into your
vagina, he reduces your body's ability to protect itself. If, at the same
time, he's also passing that bug along to you—well, it's pretty easy to
see why a woman's risk of infection is so high.

Indeed, according to the latest statistics from the Centers for Disease Control, there are an alarming 15 million new cases of sexually
transmitted diseases reported in the United States every year, most
classified into two categories:

- Infections, which are caused by bacteria and other micro-
  organisms (such as chlamydia, gonorrhea, syphilis, chancroid,
  pubic lice, yeast infections, BV, and trichomoniasis)
- Viruses, including herpes, HIV, HPV (genital warts), and hepatitis B

While the risk of either type of STD increases in proportion to the
number of sex partners you have, being monogamous doesn't guarantee protection. Indeed, some STDs can silently reside in the body for
ten, fifteen, or even twenty years without a single symptom, so you or
your partner may be infected and not even know it. For women, this
threat is even greater than for men. Studies show that symptoms of at
least one STD, chlamydia, remain silent in women up to 85 percent
of the time, as compared to just 40 percent of the time in men.

What can help is becoming familiar with the facts and information you need to keep these diseases from doing you any real harm. And in the remainder of this chapter you will find just such information about the most common sexually transmitted infections. The following chapter contains similar information about the sex viruses, or "love bugs," that can do you the most harm. Together, these two chapters offer you important guidelines that can help you enjoy sex more while protecting your health *and* your reproductive future.

The Sex Infections:
What a Woman Needs to Know

Although a wide variety of sexually transmitted infections affect women today, by far the most common are chlamydia, gonorrhea, trichomoniasis, and syphilis. While each has its own set of symptoms as well as specific treatments (and we'll get to those specifics shortly), when left untreated, all these diseases have similar consequences in common.

Indeed, beginning anywhere from a few days to a few weeks after infection, most women usually experience either cervicitis, an inflammation of the cervical canal, or urethritis (also known as nongonococcal urethritis, or NGU)—inflammation within the urethra, the tubelike structure that carries urine from the body. The good news is that when these are recognized at the early stages, generally all that's needed to stop these infections is a simple regimen of antibiotics.

When, however, any of these conditions are left untreated, even for a little while, the invading bacteria or micro-organisms can begin a dangerous ascent through your reproductive system. As they invade the upper reproductive tract, a potentially deadly condition known as pelvic inflammatory disease, or PID, can develop. According to the CDC, statistics on at least one common STD, chlamydia, show the rate of PID at about 40 percent—meaning that four out of every ten women who are infected will develop this more severe form of pelvic disease.

If this does occur, it means the inflammation can spread to your uterus (causing a condition called endometritis), fallopian tubes (causing salpingitis), or the ovaries (resulting in oophoritis). As white blood cells multiply to fight the infection, pus can form, which may later fill the fallopian tubes or various areas of the pelvic cavity, causing even more inflammation.

Although it's rare, an abscess (a pus-filled sac) can form on any of the reproductive organs. Should it rupture, another life-threatening

AN EXPERT'S OPINION ON . . .

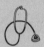

The Symptoms of PID

Could you have pelvic inflammatory disease—PID—and not know it? Experts say it's possible. Indeed, while symptoms are usually quite prominent, this is not *always* the case. Indeed, sometimes symptoms can be so slight they can easily be ignored. In some instances, there may be no symptoms at all, particularly when the infection is the result of chlamydia.

Additionally, it's also possible to mistake the symptoms of PID for something else, such as appendicitis or even the stomach flu.

According to sex health experts at the Mayo Foundation for Medical Education and Research, however, for most women the following telltale symptoms are the most obvious warning signs of PID:

- Pain in lower abdomen
- Heavy vaginal discharge, particularly with an odor
- Irregular menstrual bleeding including spotting between periods
- Pain during intercourse
- Lower back pain
- Fever
- Fatigue
- Diarrhea
- Vomiting

condition known as peritonitis can develop. In this instance, the infection can spread throughout the entire abdominal cavity as well as the pelvic region. If not treated quickly, this rare but dramatic form of PID can be so devastating to the body that death can result.

STDs and Your Fertility

Fortunately, for most women, the pain leading up to the horrific stages of PID is so encompassing that treatment is rarely delayed for any significant amount of time. And once antibiotics are administered, the infections clear fairly rapidly, allowing the life-threatening aspect of the illness to pass.

However, simply clearing a PID infection is not the end the story. Ironically, for many women, the true damage caused by STDs doesn't really start until the infection begins to heal. That's when scar tissue can develop. An overgrowth of cells that is the body's natural response to tissue damage (in this case caused by the STD), scar tissue (also known as adhesions) can begin growing almost anywhere the infection was present, including the cervix, uterus, fallopian tubes, or ovaries. Depending on where that excess tissue develops and the degree to which it forms, a number of fertility-related consequences can occur. In the fallopian tubes, for example, scar tissue can make egg transport difficult or impossible and can literally stop sperm from ever reaching an egg. In the ovary, it may block ovulation. And when scar tissue forms in the uterus, it may not be able to respond to the hormonal stimulation necessary to build the spongy lining that enables an embryo to implant and grow.

Additionally, if you do manage to get pregnant, research also shows that some sexually transmitted infections, particularly the silent infection chlamydia, can significantly increase your risk of miscarriage. In some instances, women have lost up to ten or more pregnancies before realizing they were quietly harboring this symptomless infection.

The important thing to remember is that no STD need ever progress to the stage where you experience any of these long-term consequences. Indeed, by becoming familiar with the early signs and symptoms of the most common STDs, you can seek treatment fast, and dramatically decrease your risk of any serious problems.

To help you know what to look for and the treatments that can help, use the following guide to the most common STD infections affecting women today. This, combined with the information on sexually transmitted viruses found in the next chapter, should give you a sound basis for long-term care that will not only result in a healthier, happier sex life, but also protect your fertility and your child bearing options at the same time.

The Five Most Common Sexually Transmitted Infections: What You Need To Know

#1. Chlamydia: The Silent Infection

Considered one of the newer STDs to affect both men and women on a broad scale, chlamydia is in fact one of the most frequently reported infectious diseases in the United States. Caused by the bacteria known as *Chlamydia trachomatis,* some 500,000 new cases occur each year. Because, however, the Centers for Disease Control (CDC) believes chlamydia often goes undiagnosed and untreated, the real number of those affected is likely closer to 4 million new cases annually. From 1984 through 1997, the rate of chlamydia rose from just over 3 cases to a whopping 207 cases, per 100,000 people.

While it has long been known that undiagnosed chlamydia is a leading cause of PID, the newest research gives us even more cause for concern. Reporting in the January 2000 issue of the *International Journal of Cancer,* researchers from the National Public Institute in Finland offer new evidence that infection with the chlamydia bacteria increases a woman's risk of invasive squamous cell cervical cancer. After analyzing data from some 530,000 Nordic women, the researchers found those who had antibodies to the chlamydia bacteria in their blood (indicating a past infection) were more than twice as likely to develop cervical cancer—even after the findings were adjusted for other risk factors.

Do You Have Chlamydia? How to Tell: According to experts at Planned Parenthood, the initial onset of symptoms usually occurs within one to three weeks following exposure and can include the following:

- Yellow vaginal discharge
- Pain during urination
- Persistent lower abdominal pain
- Pain during intercourse
- Spotting during periods
- Nausea and fever

It is, however, important to note that up to 75 percent of all women infected with chlamydia have no symptoms, or the signs are so subtle they can be difficult to detect. Additionally, when symptoms do appear, they can be transient, lasting from several weeks up to fifteen months and then disappearing. But while the overt symptoms may be gone, the infection is not, which means that not only can you still pass it on to someone else, but that any damage associated with this infection continues to occur, particularly in your reproductive system.

Does your partner have chlamydia? What to look for:

- A discolored penile discharge
- Noticeably painful urination

Important to note: up to 40 percent of men with chlamydia have no symptoms.

Are You at Risk? Any woman who is sexually active is at risk for chlamydia, and the younger you are, the greater your risk may be. Indeed, peak susceptibility begins around age thirteen and continues until the mid- to late twenties. Experts theorize that this may be due to the fact that younger women often have thinner vaginal mucus, which allows for a speedier transport of the bacteria through the reproductive system. Others believe that because the cervix does not fully close until a woman reaches her mid-twenties, any bacteria deposited in the vagina have a direct entry to the cervix, which makes it easier for any STD to spread through the reproductive tract. Indeed, experts at Johns Hopkins Medical Institute caution that, because the risk of this infection in young women is so high and the concurrent risk of infertility so great, all sexually active adolescents should be tested by family doctors twice a year.

And while it was once thought that women were more susceptible than men to chlamydia, researchers from the National Institute of Allergy and Infectious Diseases say this is not true. Newer, more sensitive diagnostic tests now show the rate to be nearly equal. However, the researchers do concede that studies on nearly 1,000 patients and their sexual partners treated at an STD clinic revealed that women are still more than twice as likely as men to have no symptoms of the infection, a fact that may increase their risk of more serious complications.

Since chlamydia is an STD, the behaviors that increase your risk the most are vaginal, anal, and oral sex. While it is extremely easy to pick up the disease in any of these intimate situations, you are *not likely* to get it from kissing or from sharing clothes, towels, or other inanimate objects with someone who harbors the infection.

The Tests and Treatments That Can Help: If you do experience symptoms of chlamydia or if you suspect or know you have been exposed, you should consider getting tested as soon as possible. Chlamydia has become so widespread that many STD experts suggest that you be routinely screened for this infection at least once yearly, and more often if you have multiple sex partners. Indeed, many experts consider it appropriate to be tested every time you have a new intimate partner.

Ironically, outdated or even sexist ideas about who *gets* chlamydia may mean your doctor *will not* routinely suggest testing or even bring up the subject during your exam. At least one survey of some 1,600 physicians conducted by the University of Pittsburgh found that just 32 percent of doctors would offer a chlamydia screening to a sexually active nineteen-year-old during a regular gynecological exam unless she complained of symptoms. (Surprisingly, the survey also found

AN EXPERT'S OPINION ON . . .

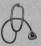

Douching and Chlamydia

While it has been long known that douching may increase the risk of certain vaginal infections, a new study of some 1,700 women published in the *Journal of Obstetrics and Gynecology* revealed it may be a particularly dangerous practice for women at risk for chlamydia. According to Dr. Delia Shoales, an epidemiologist with the University of Washington School of Public Health who conducted the new studies, women who reported douching within one year prior to the study had more than a twofold increased risk of contracting chlamydia than women who never used a douche. Dr. Shoales also discovered that the more a woman douches, the greater is her risk of infection. More specifically, the risk was more than two and half times higher for women who douched one to three times a month and nearly four times higher for women who douched four or more times a month when compared to women who did not douche.

The reason for the increase? Not only does douching change the vaginal environment, increasing susceptibility to all infections, but Dr. Shoales believes the force of the liquid inside the vagina may actually remove a protective layer of mucus in the cervix, leaving you more susceptible to infection. If you already have an infection—and remember that chlamydia may not show any symptoms—Dr. Shoales reports that the liquid may help spread your infection higher into your reproductive tract, thus increasing your risk of complications.

While some experts still question these direct links, most agree that douching in general is not necessary and should be avoided.

that pediatricians and internists were more likely to offer STD testing than family physicians or gynecologists and obstetricians, ostensibly because they may be more in touch with the fact that we are all becoming sexually active at a much younger age.) The point here is that it may be up to you to query your doctor about your need for testing.

What should you request? By the late 1990s we began to see a whole new breed of tests for chlamydia, some of which are among the easiest and the most accurate available. Of the newest ones, those thought to be the most successful, in terms of rapid, accurate diagnosis, are known as nucleic acid amplification tests. There are three such FDA-approved chlamydia tests of this type:

• PCR Amplicor *Chlamydia trachomatis* test
• LCR LCx *Chlamydia trachomatis* assay
• TMA GenProbe Amplified *Chlamydia trachomatis* assay

All three use either cervical swabs or urine samples. Studies have demonstrated that each of the tests has a sensitivity of 80 to 100 percent, as compared to 65 to 88 percent for a standard culture. This means that these new tests are nearly 30 percent more likely to correctly identify your infection.

If you test positive for chlamydia only, treatment is fast and easy. According to the latest 1998 CDC Treatment Guidelines for chlamydia, the most common antibiotics are doxycycline, azithromycin, ofloxacin, and erythromycin.

In order to ensure against reinfection, the CDC suggests that partners need to be treated as well even if they do not test positive for symptoms. Specifically, anyone with whom you have had sexual contact within sixty days needs to be tested, and your last partner needs to be tested as well, even if it has been longer than sixty days since you were sexually active.

If Left Untreated: What You Can Expect: For some women, a lack of symptoms means the diagnosis is simply missed. For others, it's a conscious effort to ignore the red flags that signal something is wrong. In either case, when chlamydia goes untreated, even for a short while, it often quickly progresses to NGU (nongonococcal urethritis), an inflammation of the tube that carries urine from the bladder, out of the body. According to experts at the McKinley Health Center of the University of Illinois, chlamydia is responsible for at least half of all cases of NGU. When this infection is left untreated, it can quickly progress to cervicitis (an infection of the cervix), which can lead to PID. Indeed, up to 40 percent of all women who contract chlamydia go on to develop PID and its fertility-related consequences.

Additionally, new studies from Wayne State University in Detroit, Michigan, found that the chlamydia organism can sometimes travel from the genitals to the joints, causing a type of inflammation known as reactive arthritis—in as little as seven days after infection. The study, which was presented at the Ninety-ninth Annual Meeting of the American Society for Microbiology, involved female guinea pigs and not humans. However, the researchers point out that the data gleaned from the guinea pig study shared a similar pathology to that seen in humans. Thus, they have reason to suspect that the infection travels the same rapid path in humans as was documented in the animal studies.

Pregnancy and Chlamydia: Because babies born to mothers with active chlamydia infections can contract the virus during delivery, treatment is essential the moment infection is diagnosed.

While two of the most common medications (doxycycline and ofloxacin) are contraindicated for use in pregnancy, the good news is experts from the Bowman Grey School of Medicine/Wake Forest University in Winston-Salem, North Carolina, have a new treatment option. Reporting in the journal *Obstetrics and Gynecology* the researchers say azithromycin is not only safe and effective when used during pregnancy, it is also well tolerated, with fewer side effects, particularly in regard to gastrointestinal complaints. Since treatment requires only one pill, it is also a more convenient option. One caveat: it can cost up to three times more than erythromycin.

If chlamydia is not treated during pregnancy, the newborn runs the risk of contracting the infection in his or her eyes or can develop a chlamydia respiratory infection, resulting in a severe type of pneumonia.

On the Horizon: A Home Test for Chlamydia: There's encouraging news that a home test for chlamydia may be on the way. In a recent report published in the *Journal of Clinical Biology,* STD experts from the University of Alabama in Birmingham say that chlamydia tests conducted at home by patients turned out to be as reliable as those administered by doctors. The study, in which half of some 300 patients used a swab to collect their own vaginal fluids, while half had their doctors use a swab to obtain samples, revealed a roughly equal number of positive results in both groups: forty-six women who took their own test had infections, while forty-four doctor-tested women had positive results.

The key, say the researchers, is the use of a highly sensitive testing method, that which uses high-tech DNA amplification to reveal the presence of infection. With this new technology now available for widespread use, the researchers say a home test for chlamydia is a reality in the very near future.

#2. Gonorrhea: The World's Oldest STD

Among the first diseases to be documented as a sexually transmitted infection, gonorrhea declined sharply following the discovery and subsequent widespread use of penicillin, beginning in the 1940s. Now, however, this STD is on the rise once again, with more than 600,000 new gonorrheal infections diagnosed in the United States each year.

Caused by the bacteria *Neisseria gonorrhoeae,* it is considered a risk for anyone who is sexually active, particularly women between the ages of twenty and thirty. And women are also more likely to contract gonorrhea from a man than the other way around. Indeed, women have a whopping 50 percent greater chance than men of contracting this infection after a single act of intercourse. Researchers theorize it may be because the gonorrhea bacteria adhere more easily to the cells lining a woman's cervix than those found inside the penal shaft. Since gonorrhea frequently coexists with chlamydia, many experts believe having this infection as well may also increase your risk. Additionally,

AN EXPERT'S OPINION ON . . .

Gonorrhea and Oral Sex

Q: Is it true you can get gonorrhea in the throat from having oral sex?

A: Yes. According to the National Institute of Allergy and Infectious Diseases, not only is it possible, it's highly likely if you perform oral sex on a partner who harbors genital gonorrhea. What's more, a partner who harbors gonorrhea in his or her throat (called pharyngeal gonorrhea) can transfer the infection to your reproductive tract if this person performs oral sex on you. Indeed, gonorrhea can thrive in the mouth, throat, rectum, and vagina, so oral sex, as well as anal and vaginal intercourse, are all considered risky.

Gonorrhea can also be spread from the genitals to the eyes via the hands, particularly if you rub your eyes directly after touching an open gonorrhea lesion.

the more sex partners you have and the more frequently you have sex, the greater your risk of infection. Statistically, any past STD infection automatically increases your risk of gonorrhea.

While some experts believe the gonorrhea bacteria can live outside the body, on inanimate objects such as toilet seats, towels, or in showers, for up to five hours, thus increasing the risk of transmission, others say this is highly unlikely. To err on the side of caution, you should consider avoiding immediate use of intimate objects used by anyone you suspect may have this infection—a family member, friend, roommate, or sex partner.

Do You Have Gonorrhea? How to Tell: For many women, gonorrhea causes few or no symptoms. When they do appear, however, they can occur as soon as three to five days after infection, or as long

AN EXPERT'S OPINION ON . . .

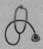

Anal Sex and Gonorrhea

Q: I've never had rectal sex, yet I ended up with a rectal gonorrheal infection. How could this happen?

A: According to experts at the National Institutes of Health, a vaginal gonorrhea infection can easily spread to the rectum, even without anal sex. By some estimates, up to 50 percent of women who contract gonorrhea vaginally also develop a coexisting rectal infection. Often symptoms of a vaginal gonorrhea infection do include rectal discomfort or discharge, as well as redness or soreness in this area. NIH experts say symptoms of rectal gonorrhea are discharge, itching, and sometimes painful bowel movements.

as three weeks after you contract the disease, with the average onset falling between seven and twenty-one days. Here is what to look for:

- An abnormally thick and creamy discharge (possibly yellow in color)
- Abnormal uterine bleeding (particularly spotting between periods)
- Pain or swelling of the labia
- Mild to moderate pelvic pain
- Burning urination

You may also experience tenderness or pain during intercourse or stool coated with mucus. In most women, the bacteria travel to the urethra (the tube leading from the bladder), causing pus in the urine, urinary frequency, and sometimes painful urination. In women who have had a hysterectomy, the urethra is frequently the primary site.

Generally oral gonorrhea has few symptoms, but you can sometimes experience a mild to moderate sore throat and some swelling in the lymph nodes in the neck.

In a very small percentage of women, gonorrhea may lead to an infection known as Fitz-Hugh-Curtis syndrome, or perihepatitis, an inflammation of the liver characterized by pain in the upper abdomen, with fever and nausea.

Does Your Partner Have Gonorrhea? What to Look For: Generally symptoms of gonorrhea are much more prevalent in men. You can look for a thick, milky discharge from the penis, and he may complain of a burning sensation during urination, usually appearing within two to seven days after exposure. Also be aware that one in five men will have no symptoms.

Is It Really Gonorrhea? **How to Know for Sure:** Although there are a variety of ways to screen for gonorrhea, many doctors rely on a test called Gram's stain, a microscopic examination of cell samples swabbed from the vagina and cervix, which is done in your doctor's office. Results are usually immediate. Some newer studies, however, have shown that this method could miss up to 60 percent of the infections in women. Thus many experts now recommend a culture as the most reliable test. Here, cell samples swabbed from your vagina or cervix (taken during your office visit) are sent to a laboratory to be grown for up to two days. This test will help determine the exact type of bacterium causing your infection. However, don't be surprised if your doctor performs both tests. Many physicians believe this is the only way to obtain a truly accurate diagnosis.

Although there are newer and faster testing techniques (including a process called direct immunofluorescence, and indirect enzyme immunoassays), they are expensive, and studies show they may be no more reliable than a standard culture.

Treatments That Can Help: In the past penicillin was always the treatment of choice for gonorrhea. Now, however, up to 25 percent of all strains of these bacteria are penicillin resistant, plus this drug has no

IMPORTANT WARNING

Since the late 1990s several strains of gonorrhea have emerged that are resistant to many of the common antibiotics used for treatment. Although the percentage of resistant strains in the United States is still considered small, the CDC reports documented outbreaks, mostly in the western states. Abroad, these tougher strains have been found in Hong Kong, the Philippines, Australia, Canada, and the United Kingdom. If your symptoms do not clear within seven to ten days after treatment, talk to your doctor about more advanced testing to identify your exact strain of gonorrhea and the antibiotics that work specifically on that strain.

Although most of the treatments for gonorrhea require seven full days of medication, there remain some, particularly injections, that require only one dose. However, the infection still takes a full seven days to clear from the body. Thus experts say to avoid intercourse for at least seven to ten days after treatment begins, even if you and your partner are both being treated simultaneously. You may also want to avoid both alcohol and caffeine during treatment, which may help to reduce some of the urinary symptoms, particularly pain or burning upon urination.

effect on chlamydia, which often coexists with the gonorrhea bacteria in the majority of women. For those reasons the CDC now suggests that a variety of newer antibiotics may be more effective. Among the most popular for confirmed cases of gonorrhea are cephalosporin antibiotics (such as cefixime and cephalexin) and a group of medications known as fluoroquinolones (drugs like ofloxacin, ciprofloxacin, and norfloxacin). Usually administered orally or by injection, these drugs are prescribed along with oral doses of doxycycline, azithromycin, or erythromycin in an attempt to kill the chlamydia infection.

If Left Untreated: What You Can Expect: For some women, the only complication stemming from their gonorrhea infection will be a mild form of cervicitis or urethritis (also known as NGU), both of which are easily treated with antibiotics.

According to the NIH, however, the most prevalent complication of gonorrhea is PID, with the resulting scar tissue often a major cause of infertility. Additionally, because gonorrhea often rapidly moves through the reproductive tract to the fallopian tubes, when left untreated it can also be a major cause of tubal damage—and still another cause of infertility.

Additionally, up to 3 percent of patients also develop what is called a disseminated infection. Here, the gonorrhea bacteria spread through the blood, causing a variety of problems. These can include a type of infection-related arthritis or tendonitis, primarily affecting the knees, elbows, ankles, and wrists, as well as endocarditis (inflammation of the heart) and meningitis (infection of the fluid surrounding the brain and spinal cord). Gonorrhea that is transmitted to the eyes can cause a form of the inflammation known as conjunctivitis.

Because symptoms of gonorrhea in women can be subtle or even nonexistent, you must always be checked for this infection if your partner is diagnosed or even if he exhibits symptoms. The CDC recommends that both partners always be treated simultaneously for both gonorrhea and chlamydia, even if only one partner tests positive for infection.

Pregnancy and Gonorrhea: According to the CDC, while a gonorrhea infection during pregnancy won't cause your baby any harm (it can't cross the placental barrier and infect your baby), it must be treated prior to delivery, or it can be passed on during the birthing process. The most susceptible area is your baby's eyes, and in the past, some infants born to mothers with gonorrhea have been blinded at birth by this infection. This is rare today, thanks to state laws that require all newborns to routinely receive eye drops immediately after birth, whether or not the mother is known to have gonorrhea.

If you do receive treatment prior to delivery, then what you *can* take, according to the CDC, is ceftriaxone—and if chlamydia is also suspected, co-treatment with erythromycin can help. You must, however, avoid treatment with both fluoroquinolones and tetracycline, because neither is considered safe during pregnancy. Remember: never keep your symptoms or your suspicions from your doctor. Diagnosis and treatment are necessary to ensure both your health and your baby's.

#3. Trichomoniasis:
The Sexually Transmitted Vaginitis

A microscopic protozoan organism known as *T. vaginalis* is the culprit behind this extremely common infection, which can live in the vagina for up to fifteen years or longer without a single symptom. Men can also silently harbor this organism in their urethra and be infected without ever knowing it.

With or without symptoms, however, this infection can still be passed on during intimate contact, which is one reason behind the high rate of infection. Indeed, according to the CDC, approximately 3 million new cases of trichomoniasis are diagnosed in the United States every year, with 176 million cases yearly worldwide. Since trichomoniasis can remain silent in the body for so many years before causing any symptoms, experts suggest the actual number of those who are affected yearly may be much higher.

Although there are few complications associated with this infection, new studies have shown that even when left untreated for an extended period of time, it may increase a woman's risk of contracting HIV, if she has sex with an infected partner at the time she also harbors trichomoniasis.

While all sexually active women are at risk for this STD, the more sex partners you have, the greater your risk. And while vaginal intercourse is the primary mode of transmission, there have been isolated medical reports of infection from contaminated toilet seats, washcloths, bathwater, and shared clothing, although none of these possibilities has been scientifically confirmed in a study.

Do You Have Trichomoniasis? How to Tell: One of the most confusing aspects of trichomoniasis is that when symptoms do appear, they are often confused with those of a urinary infection, including burning during urination, urinary frequency, and an irritated vulva. Often even doctors can misdiagnose this infection, particularly if they offer an opinion based on a telephone consultation only.

However, according to the CDC, you can avoid confusion by taking note of a frothy yellow-green or gray discharge, particularly if it has a strong odor. It can develop as soon as three to five days after becoming infected—or take five, ten, or more years to develop. Some women may also experience itching as well as painful sex, which do not normally occur with a urinary tract infection.

Does Your Partner Have Trichomoniasis? What to Look For:
Unfortunately, most men have few, if any, symptoms. When signs do appear, look for the head of the penis to be red and inflamed, and your partner may indicate discomfort during urination. Often, however, these initial symptoms will clear on their own, usually within several weeks. This does not mean the infection has cleared from his

---

SEX, TRICHOMONIASIS, AND DIVORCE

Q: My husband and I have been married, and I thought faithful to each other, for eleven years. Now I suddenly come down with trichomoniasis, and my husband was diagnosed as well. He swears he's not fooling around, and I know I'm not. So where did this infection come from. Is he lying?

A: Because trichomoniasis can lie dormant in the body for many years, it is often difficult to ascertain when and from whom you or your husband contracted this infection. Either one of you could well have had it before you even met and then passed it on during your relationship, without ever knowing it. So relax, believe him, and make certain you both get treated. If the infection occurs again, however, call your doctor and have a serious talk with your husband.

body. Quite the contrary. Men can easily transmit trichomoniasis to a woman, even if they have not had any symptoms for months or even years. Indeed, without treatment, it is highly likely the infection will remain silently in a man's body for an indefinite period of time.

The Tests and Treatments That Can Help: Your doctor will suspect trichomoniasis if, during your pelvic exam, he or she discovers a "strawberry" cervix—small, red dots that appear on the entrance to the uterus, and usually occur from a small amount of bleeding caused by the infection. Trichomoniasis can also sometimes be detected on a routine Pap smear, which can come back with a reading of irregular cells. Indeed, experts say that if you do receive a report of an irregular Pap smear, talk to your doctor about treatment for trichomoniasis for at least seven to ten days, to be followed by another Pap smear. Often you may find that once the infection clears, your Pap smear will be normal, and you'll be able to avoid extensive, invasive testing for cervical cancer.

To be tested specifically for trichomoniasis, your doctor will take a sample of your vaginal fluids, place it in saltwater solution, and view it under a microscope, which should show the presence of the tiny protozoans.

According to the latest CDC treatment guidelines, if trichomoniasis is diagnosed, the treatment of choice for both men and women is oral metronidazole (Flagyl, Metryl, Protostat). It is generally administered either in one large dose of 2 grams or 500 mg twice a day for seven days. In either case, the infection won't clear from your body for the full seven days.

Although the medication does work for most people, recently it has been noted that some strains of *T. vaginalis* have become highly resistant to treatment, often requiring larger doses or continued repeated treatments. In some instances, the infections do not respond to treatment at all. When this is the case, new studies conducted at the Temple University Vaginitis Referral Center have found a topical antibiotic cream known as paromycin may help. Reporting in the May 1998 *Clinical Infectious Diseases,* the researchers confirmed the effectiveness of this treatment, which worked even in particularly stubborn cases. Additionally, it has been medically reported that

AN EXPERT'S OPINION ON . . .

The Pill and Trichomoniasis

Q: I have been diagnosed with trichomoniasis four times in six years. My doctor suggested that birth control pills might help me avoid future infections. Is this true?

A: It could very well be. New studies conducted at University of Minnesota and Hennepin County Medical Center in Minneapolis found that the estrogen component found in most birth control pills may offer some protective effects against trichomoniasis, particularly when compared to contraceptives containing only progesterone.

Reporting at an annual Interscience Conference on Antimicrobial Agents and Chemotherapy, the researchers revealed that 47 percent of women who took a progesterone-only pill tested positive for trichomoniasis, compared to just 7 percent of the women who used a combination estrogen-progesterone pill. Additionally, 47 percent of women who used no contraceptives were found to harbor trichomoniasis.

But while birth control pills may help you, experts say make certain to also have your partner checked and treated, since he or she may be the source of your recurring infections.

some women have found some symptom relief (but not a cure) using the intravaginal wash Aci-Jel.

Pregnancy and Trichomoniasis: The latest studies show that, when present during pregnancy, trichomoniasis can increase the risk of premature rupture of the membranes, leading to premature labor and early delivery. There is also some evidence that this infection may contribute to the incidence of low-birthweight babies, usually the result of a premature delivery.

For this reason, you should be screened for trichomoniasis and treated prior to conceiving. If the infection is contracted during pregnancy or a previously undetected infection begins causing symptoms, studies show you must avoid treatment with metronidazole during the first trimester. It is, however, safe to use after the twentieth week of pregnancy. Usually one 2 gram dose is the recommended amount. Also, check with your doctor as to whether the new paromycin antibiotic cream would be right for you.

Finally, it's important to note that some fertility experts believe the *Trichomonas* parasite is associated with changes in the vaginal environment that can contribute to conception difficulties or increase the risk of miscarriage. In men, it can attach to sperm and affect transport, decreasing motility and making it more difficult to reach the egg. If you are having problems getting pregnant or maintaining a pregnancy, you and your partner should consider being tested for trichomoniasis, even if no symptoms are present.

#4. Syphilis: The STD That's Making a Comeback

Caused by tiny, spiral-shaped bacteria known as *Treponema pallidum,* as recently as the 1970s syphilis was nearly extinct. Then a surprising upswing in the number of cases in the 1980s and 1990s caught researchers and doctors by surprise. Although no one is certain what was behind the sudden dramatic increase—there are some 120,000 new cases every year—according to the CDC, not only have rates gone up, women are among the most prevalent victims, now affected twice as often as men. African American women are at greatest risk—they are seven times more likely to contract syphilis than all other races of women combined.

Although those at greatest risk are women with partners who are infected, you may be surprised to learn that there is only a 30 percent chance of contracting syphilis after an intimate encounter with an infected man. However, risks do escalate if the infection is in the early stages, when lesions are active. After one year, when the disease goes into the latent stage, transmission is more unlikely.

AN EXPERT'S OPINION ON . . .

Testing for Syphilis

Q: A man I was sleeping with about a year ago has just now been diagnosed with syphilis. Should I be worried, and do I need to be tested? What about my current partner? Should he be tested as well?

A: According to the CDC, partners are considered at risk if they have had sex:
- Within three months, plus the duration of symptoms, during the early, active stage
- Within six months, plus the duration of symptoms, during the secondary stage
- Within one year of the onset of the latent stage

In addition to intercourse, there is some evidence that syphilis may be transmitted by deep kissing or, more rarely, from nonsexual contact with an active lesion. Although extremely rare, it may also be transmitted via a blood transfusion.

Could You Have Syphilis? What to Look For: One of the most misleading factors about syphilis is the way in which symptoms occur. More specifically, many people do not realize how dramatically the signs can change during the various stages or that they usually disappear spontaneously between stages.

When diagnosed *early* on, syphilis is a relatively harmless disease that is quickly and easily cured. If symptoms are ignored, they will disappear on their own—but the disease does not. Indeed, it progresses to the latent stage, where it can remain in the body for up to twenty years or even longer, without a single symptom. Then, suddenly, without warning, it transgresses to what is called the tertiary stage, with severe complications capable of affecting the heart, brain, eyes, and ears. Problems associated with this stage include heart disease, dementia, lack of coordination, blindness, hearing loss, mental illness, paralysis, and eventually death.

To avoid all these complications, look for these early signs, appearing approximately ten days to three weeks after infection. According to the CDC they are:

- A painless ulcer (called a chancre) on the vagina or vulva. It usually disappears within five weeks with or without treatment.
- Within two to eight weeks after the sore appears, the syphilis bacteria invade the bloodstream, causing a number of flulike symptoms, including malaise, fatigue, sore throat, joint pain, and headache.
- A flushed, flat, red rash usually appears on the hands and soles of the feet, also within the two- to eight-week period.

All of these symptoms also clear, usually within two to ten weeks, with or without treatment. Although the symptoms may disappear on their own, the infection does not; it is still considered active and may be transmitted.

Does Your Partner Have Syphilis? What to Look For: A blister or open sore on the penis or scrotum, as well as a flat red rash on the hands and feet is often the sign of an early-stage infection.

The Tests and Treatments That Can Help: If you suspect or know you have been exposed to syphilis, and especially if you already have experienced the characteristic vulvar sore, you must be tested right away. Currently, there are two basic diagnostics, both painless and relatively easy. The first test examines cell samples taken from your suspicious chancre and looks for the presence of the infecting micro-organism itself; the second test looks for immune system antibodies that form in the blood after infection. The method of testing is usually determined by the stage of infection at the time of testing. Generally, however, these are your options:

- Early stage: The dark-field examination, a method of examining the chancres through a microscope for an on-site diagnosis.
- Later stages: One of four basic blood tests: Venereal Disease Research Laboratory (VDRL) test; fluorescent treponemal antibody (FTA) absorption test; rapid plasma reagin (RPR) test; treponemal hemagglutination (TPHA) assay.

The VDRL and RPR are fast, inexpensive, and easy, but they can show a false positive, indicating syphilis where none exists. Often a doctor likes to confirm the results of these tests with the FTA and TPHA, which detect syphilis antibodies (proteins made by the immune system in response to infection).

If syphilis is diagnosed, don't panic: it's easily treated. The most commonly prescribed, and consequently the most effective, treatment is penicillin. The CDC recommends a single dose of 2.4 million units of penicillin G benzathine. In the event of a penicillin allergy, tetracycline or doxycycline can sometimes be used. Additionally, if you have been exposed to syphilis, it may be wise to get treated even if your test results are negative. The CDC guidelines are as follows:

- Consider treatment if you have been intimate with an infected person for any length of time up to ninety days prior to diagnosis.
- Definitely seek treatment if you have been intimate with an infected person any time after diagnosis.

Pregnancy and Syphilis: Because the risk of transmitting syphilis from mother to baby is so great, the CDC recommends that every woman be screened at least once, either right before or during her pregnancy. Indeed, each year more than 3,000 cases of congenital syphilis (transmitted from mother to baby) are diagnosed, with some studies indicating that the more recent the mother's syphilis infection, the greater is the risk of passing the disease to her baby. Death of the fetus or newborn occurs in up to 40 percent of all pregnant women who remain untreated for syphilis. The CDC also recommends that any woman who delivers a stillborn child at more than twenty weeks of gestation should be tested for syphilis and that no infant should be allowed to leave the hospital unless the mother has been tested for this disease at least once during her pregnancy.

According to the 1998 CDC guidelines for STDs, treatment of syphilis during pregnancy should be the penicillin regimen that is appropriate for the specific stage of the disease at diagnosis. Ultrasound exams can be used to help detect signs of fetal infection and may also help determine treatment regimens.

Treatment during the second half of pregnancy could increase the risk of premature labor and the baby's risk of fetal distress, so the earlier you are diagnosed and treated, the better it is for you *and* your baby.

Taking Charge of Your Sexual Health: What to Do

The information presented on STD infections in this chapter, together with the latest data on sexually transmitted viruses found in the next chapter, should give you a strong basis from which to work with your doctor to help encourage a healthier, happier, more fulfilling sex life. If, however, you are still planning to rely solely on your doctor to detect a sexually transmitted infection during a routine gynecologic exam, there are a few words of warning you must hear.

First, many infections simply don't show up during the course of routine care. Moreover, there's a good possibility your doctor won't even broach the subject of testing unless you bring it up. Indeed, during a recent Gallup poll, more than 50 percent of the women queried said their doctors never questioned them about their sexual practices or their risk of disease. Likewise, 70 percent of the women participating in a 1999 survey conducted by the Kaiser Family Foundation in conjunction with the *Los Angeles Times* and *Latina* magazine said their doctors *never* asked them about their level of sexual activity, their number of partners, or if they were monogamous. The same number said they were never questioned about their sexual history or whether they used condoms.

If you want to ensure the best possible V zone care, you must make a concerted effort to talk to your doctor about your sexual health, whether or not he or she brings the subject up. This should include

TALKING POINTS

Admittedly, talking to your doctor about your sex life *can* be uncomfortable, and bringing up the topic yourself can make things even more difficult. This can be true whether your physician is a man or a woman. To make things easier, experts suggest reducing tensions by easing your way into the subject rather than hitting it head on—for example:

• If you can't say: "I've just slept with another new partner."

Try: "I've met someone new, and I'm really enjoying the relationship. But I do have a few health concerns."

• If you can't say: "I think my boyfriend is sleeping around, and I'm worried."

Try: "Is there any way I can tell if my boyfriend might have been exposed to an STD outside our relationship?"

• If you can't say: "I've been unfaithful to my husband, and I need an STD test."

Try: "I may have been exposed to an STD outside of my marriage, and I'd like to be tested."

• If you can't say: "I think my boyfriend is having sex with another man, and I want an HIV test."

Try: "I'm not certain about my boyfriend's social activities when I'm not around; an HIV test would really ease my mind."

If your doctor is at all sensitive to your needs, which he or she should be, then all you need do is *hint* about the subject of sex, and it should open the topic for a relaxed and easy discussion. If it doesn't, consider finding a new physician.

not only a discussion of any symptoms of STD infections that you might have noticed, but also the extent of your sexual relationships, including the number of partners, their sex, and, if applicable, the number and sex of any other partners they might have. If you are very active sexually, be diligent about requesting regular testing for some of the most common STDs, and if your doctor won't cooperate, find one who will. It's that simple and that important.

If you are diagnosed with an infection, don't panic, but do insist on the most progressive and proactive care. Then be certain to participate in all follow-up exams and continue to be tested regularly. Once you have had one STD, your risk for contracting others automatically increases.

It Can Happen To You:
Some Final Advice

If you're like most other women, you probably believe all this STD advice *doesn't* really apply to you. Indeed, a 1998 survey conducted by the Kaiser Family Foundation and *Glamour* magazine found only about 2 percent of women aged eighteen to forty-four considered themselves at high risk for contracting a sexually transmitted disease. A similar survey found that only about 15 percent of women were concerned enough to talk to their doctor about being tested for an STD.

Reality Check I: The CDC reminds us that one in every four Americans will get an STD in their lifetime, and two-thirds will be affected before they reach age twenty-five.

What's that you say? You only sleep with men who confirm they are healthy?

Reality Check II: According to that 1998 Kaiser Family Foundation/*Glamour* magazine survey, while *some* men tell their partners if they have a sexually transmitted disease, most only do so *after* they have already had sex. And many never bother to tell their partners at all.

CHAPTER EIGHT

The Love Bugs

A Guide to Sexually Transmitted Viruses

If you've ever had a common cold, then you've already experienced a virus. There are, in fact, hundreds of varieties, from simple organisms—like those that cause a case of the sniffles or mild stomach flu—to ones that cause complex, even life-threatening illnesses.

In terms of your *sexual* health, however, there are just four viruses about which you need be concerned: genital herpes (HSV), human papilloma virus (HPV), human immunodeficiency virus (HIV), and hepatitis B (HBV). Although each one is different, with vastly different consequences, once in the body, all viruses react in a similar way.

Indeed, the main goal of every virus is to reproduce itself. In order to do that, it needs a healthy, noninfected normal cell. So regardless of how you contract a virus—whether it involves sexual contact or not—once inside the body, the first step is always to find that healthy cell and make its way inside. As soon as it does, the virus begins releasing the chemical information necessary to reproduce itself. In a sense, its turns your healthy cell into a little virus factory, producing and then releasing copies of itself into your bloodstream. In turn, each copied virus finds its own healthy host cell and begins the same process. Soon thousands of viral cells are cloned and busily reproducing themselves over and over again.

Depending on what the specific virus is, this duplication and infection process can last anywhere from a few days (in the case of the common cold) to indefinitely, as is the case with HIV, the virus that causes AIDS. Essentially, most antiviral medications work by attempting to halt this replication process.

Although some viruses, like that which causes the common cold, burn out on their own, this is not the case for the four major sexually transmitted viruses. Indeed, once contracted, these viruses stay with you for life. And although the symptoms may not always be present and there are treatments available to help reduce what you do experience, once you have a viral STD, you always run the risk of passing it on to someone else.

For this reason it's extremely important that you learn the risk factors for each of these four viruses, including what you can do to protect yourself. In the event that you do contract one of these illnesses, recognizing the signs and getting help early on is one of the best ways not only to minimize your suffering, but also to reduce your chances of passing the virus on to someone else. In the case of HIV, early diagnosis and treatment could extend your life by a significant margin, sometimes adding twenty or more healthy years.

To this end, you can use the following guide to help ensure that you do know all the essentials about the four most common viral STDs, including how to protect yourself from harm.

Virus #1:
The Human Papilloma Virus

Can you remember getting tiny warts on the tips of your fingers when you were a child—the kind we always thought came from touching frogs? If so, then you already have some experience with the human papilloma virus (HPV), an organism that causes, among other things, warts. Indeed, there are some seventy different strains of HPV, and what you might not know is that at least some can be transmitted sexually. Two in particular—HPV 6 and HPV 11—cause genital warts, growths that can be similar to what used to appear on your fingers, only this time they develop in and around your V zone. Most often they occur when you have intimate contact with a partner who also harbors the virus. Because it is so contagious—viral cells can easily shed from the warts to the surrounding skin—often the only thing an infected partner need do is touch his genitals and then touch yours—and transmission takes place. HPV can also be transmitted through nonsexual contact. For example, if you use a toilet moments after someone with warts, it's possible to pick up the virus.

But while the warts can be a painful and unsightly nuisance, you may be surprised to learn that they pose no real danger to your health. Far more lethal are the more than one dozen other strains of HPV that by and large cause no visible symptoms but have been linked to a significant risk of V zone cancers. Indeed, a six-year study published in 1999 issues of both the *Journal of Pathology* and the British medical journal *Lancet* revealed that at least one or more strains of HPV are present in virtually all cases of cervical cancer—an astounding 99.7 percent.

As frightening a finding as this is, it doesn't even tell the whole story. Research has also shown that strains of HPV appear to be connected to cancers throughout the entire V zone, including the vagina, vulva, and the anus. In one 1998 study conducted at the Institute for Epidemiological Cancer Research in Scandinavia, some 35 percent of genital cancers were traced to several strains of HPV, including 16, 18, and 22. The women at highest risk for vulvar cancer harbored HPV 16, which was also associated with some cases of vaginal cancer. Researchers also found HPV strains 16, 18 or 33 present in many anal cancers, with the highest number of cases attributed to HPV 16.

This research supported the findings of a 1997 Scandinavian study published in the *New England Journal of Medicine*. Here, data on some 1,500 Danish and Swedish patients revealed that up to 84 percent of those with anal cancer tested positive for HPV, particularly HPV 16.

Although women seemed to be more affected by these viruses, it wasn't long before researchers realized that men too are at risk. In 1997 scientists from the National Cancer Institute used high-tech DNA-HPV tests to screen stored blood samples taken from some 50,000 participants in a thirty-year health study that began in 1959. Preliminary analysis has shown that men infected with HPV 16 were up to five times more likely to develop prostate cancer.

Currently, an expert panel from the World Health Organization

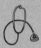

AN EXPERT'S OPINION ON . . .

HPV and HIV: An Important New Link

Can strains of HPV increase your risk of contracting HIV, the virus that causes AIDS? Some studies indicate it's possible. Research published in the *New England Journal of Medicine* in 1998 revealed that women who were HIV positive were up to seven times more likely to have a persistent HPV infection. What's more, the lower a woman's T-cell count (an indication of the stage of her HIV infection), the higher her risk of recurring, ongoing infection. Whether the HPV came before the HIV was not immediately known; however, other studies have shown that women with HIV do have a high rate of cervical cancer, another factor that links these two viruses together.

Will all women who contract HPV get AIDS? Certainly not. But if you are exposed to the virus, having HPV may increase the risk that you will become infected.

suggests that certain strains of HPV—particularly 16, 18, 31, and 33—are, in fact, so dangerous to human health that they should be labeled carcinogenic.

Are You at Risk?

If you're like most other women, you're probably thinking that you're not really in all that much danger and that your risk for HPV is probably low. But underestimating your vulnerability could be a mistake. According to the CDC, more than 24 million Americans harbor at least one strain of HPV, with more than 1 million new cases diagnosed every year, many in women under age forty.

Studies published in the *New England Journal of Medicine* as recently as 1998 revealed that sexually active college-aged women have one of the *highest* rates of HPV infection: up to 46 percent are thought to carry the virus. Similar rates of infection were found among the more than 600 women who enrolled in the National Institute of Allergy and Infectious Diseases (NIAID) study of HPV. According to researchers from the Albert Einstein College of Medicine in the Bronx, New York, white women had the highest rate of disease. Some 57 percent had HPV, compared to 13 percent of Hispanic women, 12 percent of black women, and 18 percent of other combined ethnic groups.

In addition to the factors that increase the risk of many STDs—including frequent vaginal and anal intercourse, multiple sex partners, and a high intake of alcohol (which may lower immunity, as well as lowering inhibitions and increasing the risk of casual sex)—there are also some specific aspects of the V zone anatomy that put women at special risk for HPV. Because the virus thrives in warm, moist environments, the V zone is the perfect nesting ground. If you also have any form of vaginitis at the time of exposure, even that which is caused by a simple yeast infection, studies show the natural increase in vaginal secretions can also increase your risk of HPV.

Now if you're thinking that all you have to do to avoid this virus is to make certain your partner isn't sporting any genital warts, remember that the most *lethal* strains of HPV may have no symptoms of any kind. You should also be aware that studies have shown that genetic material from the human papilloma virus has been found in semen, indicating it may be present in all bodily fluids.

Could You Have HPV? How to Tell

When it comes to diagnosing HPV, the ease with which your infection can be verified depends a lot on the strain of the virus you are carrying. If you have contracted HPV 6 or 11, it's likely you have developed genital warts, which can appear anywhere from four weeks to six months or longer after exposure. According to experts at the Mayo Foundation for Medical Education and Research, when they do develop, they are often flat, oval-shaped growths that closely resemble the warts that grow on your fingers. They can also start out as tiny red or pink bumps about the size of a grain of rice and then later blossom into large, fleshy, cauliflower-shaped growths, usually within several weeks. Sometimes they can grow to 3 inches or larger in size and even

AN EXPERT'S OPINION ON . . .

New Warts and Old Lovers

Q: I was recently diagnosed with genital warts, and when I asked my doctor if it was likely that I caught it from my husband, he said I could just as easily have caught it from someone else. I was insulted. I don't cheat on my husband. How could my doctor even assume that I did!

A: While your doctor could have been a bit more diplomatic in his phrasing, what he was likely referring to was the fact that HPV can lie dormant in the body for many years, without any visible symptoms—which means you may have contracted the virus from *anyone* in your past. Dr. Karl R. Buetner, a California dermatologist who helped develop the 1999 AMA guidelines on HPV, recently told the journal *Skin Allergy News* that "the incubation period can be months to years, it may not be the most recent love."

This advice, by the way, goes for your husband as well as for you. If, in fact, it turns out you did contract HPV from him, he could have contracted the original infection long before he knew you.

While doctors aren't certain why some people develop the warts right away and others do not, recent studies point to the immune system as the link. When for some reason your system has a temporary dip in protection—due to another illness or sometimes just fatigue or stress—your defenses go down and the warts can appear.

Another possible explanation is that you had the warts all along but that they were confined to your cervix, which would have been hard for you to see. Technically, of course, a gynecologist should have spotted any previously existing warts, but that often depends on how thorough and how observant your doctor is. Sometimes warts can be very difficult to spot without specific testing.

interfere with the ability to walk or sit. Frequently they can cause intense itching or burning as well.

Generally genital warts are diagnosed by clinical observation, although sometimes, when a growth is very small, your doctor may elect to perform a biopsy. Here, a small sampling of cells is scraped from the surface of the wart and then analyzed for HBV 6 or 11.

Much more difficult to diagnose are subclinical HPV infections. Although they are the most dangerous form, they present no obvious outward signs. For many years doctors were forced to rely solely on the Pap smear (see Chapter 1) as the main HPV diagnostic tool. While the screening couldn't detect the virus, it could indicate if an abnormality was present. If, in fact, the Pap smear came back from the laboratory as abnormal, the next step was a colposcopy (an internal examination using a specially designed microscope) followed by a cervical biopsy. Only then could doctors know for certain if a woman had HPV and, more important, cervical cancer.

Now, however, a brand-new test is changing the way the diagnosis is made. Indeed, when a Pap smear does indicate that something is amiss or even if your doctor wants to double-check the diagnosis of genital warts, a new DNA screening can help, while eliminating unnecessary invasive diagnostic procedures. Approved by the FDA in 1999, the test is called Hybrid Capture II, and it relies on sophisticated DNA technology to identify the presence of HPV molecules in cervical cells and classify the virus as to the exact type. It can, say experts, identify all thirteen of the deadliest strains of HPV.

So just how good is this new technology? When combined with a Pap smear, studies on some 1,000 women conducted at the Kaiser Permanente Division of Research in Oakland, California, found it had an overall accuracy rate of 96.9 percent in terms of detecting both HPV and cervical cancer at the earliest stage. However, the test itself is still being scrutinized as part of a large-scale, five-year National Cancer Institute study that won't be completed for several more years. You should also know that the latest results—two studies published in the January 2000 issue of the *Journal of the American Medical Association*—revealed the HPV test may yield a higher rate of false positives than the Pap smear—nearly double the amount. As such the test remains approved only for use with a Pap smear.

HPV AND MEN

Q: I just started sleeping with a new partner and I noticed some sort of growth on his scrotum. He said it's a birthmark—kind of like a scar—but I'm not so sure. Could it be an STD?

A: If the scar looks flat, oval and flesh colored, or large and cauliflower shaped, he could have HPV. When warts do appear in men, they generally grow on the shaft of the penis or the scrotum, as well as on the glans penis and sometimes the urethra. If you're not sure what you see, tell him what you suspect, and ask if he would consent to a test. If that's not possible, keep checking yourself for signs of infection, and do share your feelings about your partner's body with your doctor. If there is any question he could have HPV, you need to be tested right away.

That said, many doctors are already recommending that the new test be automatically combined with a Pap smear for routine testing of all sexually active women, and at least some say that before long, they expect the HPV test alone to become the gold standard for cervical cancer screening, particularly in women over age thirty-five.

Condoms and HPV: Will They Help?

One of the reasons this disease is rampant is that it is so easily passed on during intimate contact. According to experts at the Mayo Foundation, that contact *doesn't have to include intercourse.* That's because the viral cells, as well as the warts, can be present anywhere in a man's P zone—his testicles, his anal area, and even his thighs. The virus is then passed on by skin-to-skin contact, particularly through microsurgical tears and abrasions that occur during sexual activity.

So, while condoms can cut down the risk of transmission (and they should always be used for matters of safety concerning other STDs), they cannot give you 100 percent protection from HPV.

If your partner knows he has this virus, talk to your doctor *before*

AN EXPERT'S OPINION ON . . .

Oral Sex and HPV

Q: Is it safe to perform oral sex on a man with genital warts?

A: If by "safe" you mean that you won't catch the virus, the answer is no. According to California dermatologist Dr. Karl Buetner reporting in *Skin Allergy News,* there is a small but definite risk of developing warts in your mouth or throat as a result of oral sex. Likewise, if you have HPV in your vagina and your partner performs oral sex on you, he can develop HPV warts in his mouth or throat. And remember that even if you don't directly touch the warts with your mouth, you can still pick up the viral cells, which shed onto the nearby skin.

starting or continuing the intimate relationship—with or without condoms.

If You Have HPV: What You Can Do

Because HPV is a virus, there is no cure. And in the case of subclinical HPV, there really is no treatment other than what would be prescribed in the event that cervical cancer was also diagnosed. If, however, you harbor the strains of HPV related to genital warts, according to the CDC, one or more of the following treatments may help.

Trichloroacetic Acid (TCA). Applied directly to the warts, this topical preparation destroys the growths by chemically burning them.

Generally this preparation should be applied by a physician and may cause some burning or pain for several minutes following appli-

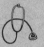

AN EXPERT'S OPINION ON . . .

How Long Is Too Long for HPV Treatment?

Q: I've been receiving TCA as treatment for genital warts for over twelve weeks, and they are not going away. Should it take this long to work, and can it be combined with some other drug to get better results? My doctor doesn't seem to want to try anything else.

A: According to the latest CDC treatment guidelines for HPV, warts should significantly improve within three treatments. With TCA, they should be completely gone within six treatments. If they are not, you should consider moving on to a different therapy. If your doctor is not familiar with other treatments, consider seeking help at an STD clinic. Often these specialized medical centers have the most experience and offer the greatest number of treatment options. Generally there is no evidence that combining treatments for HPV increases the effectiveness or speed of relief, and it could increase complications.

cation. Usually TCA must be repeated at one- to two-week intervals for several weeks, or until the warts disappear. Dusting your genitals with sodium bicarbonate (baking soda) after each treatment may help neutralize excess acid and reduce local irritation.

Podophyllin Resin. A topical application applied directly to the growth, it encourages a chemical coagulation of protein that causes the wart to shrivel and die. Treatment should always be administered by a doctor.

A reportedly painful treatment, it may continue to burn and cause discomfort for up to four days afterward. Generally, however, you probably won't need more than one or two treatments to destroy warts. According to the CDC, washing off the chemicals within one to four hours afterward can reduce vulvar irritation. So will air-drying the genitals before you get dressed. If burning is significant, a dusting with bicarbonate of soda will offer some relief. Although some toxicity has been associated with this treatment, you should be safe as long as your doctor limits the amount used per application to no more than .5 ml.

Interferon. One of the newer prescription drugs for HPV, this preparation is either injected directly into each wart or administered systemically by injection into the buttocks or arm. Treatments should be repeated several times a week for up to three weeks.

Interferon has been shown not only to have antiviral properties, but, because it appears to stimulate the immune system, it may mobilize the body's own forces to help destroy the warts. However, this treatment is associated with a high rate of adverse effects, and since it requires numerous doctor visits, it may be more expensive to use.

Imiquimod (Aldara). The newest HPV treatment, this topical cream can be safely used on a regular basis for up to sixteen weeks, with most warts disappearing within eight to ten weeks. It can be administered for the first time by a physician or by the patient, and treatment can then be continued at home.

Believed to cause the least irritation and discomfort of any of the topical wart treatments, there is also evidence it may destroy strains of HPV that cause cervical cancer. According to research conducted at McGill University in Montreal, Canada, the molecule that makes up this treatment has antiviral properties. Although it won't kill HPV, it has been shown to stimulate a person's own immune system into recognizing the virus cells and destroying them. Aldara was also shown to be effective in patients who smoke, use birth control pills, or drink alcohol—all factors that have been known to reduce the effectiveness of other HPV treatments.

Podofilox Gel or Solution. Using a cotton swab, you can apply this treatment yourself, usually twice a day for three days, followed by four days of no treatment. This treatment cycle usually must be repeated four times before all warts clear.

Podofilox should be used only on warts under 10 centimeters in size, and you should never use more than .5 ml in a twenty-four-hour period. It's also a good idea to have your doctor administer the first dose, so you can get a sense of how much to apply. You may experience mild to moderate pain, or localized irritation following each treatment.

Cryotherapy or Freezing. During this treatment your doctor will apply a chemical called liquid nitrogen directly to each wart. This causes a freezing sensation, followed by throbbing, and finally burning, as the area begins to "thaw." Within one to two days, blisters develop, which usually clear within two weeks.

It is important that the blisters that form after treatment are not broken and that the genital area be kept very clean and dry throughout the healing process. It's also important that your doctor be an expert in working with this solution. Often a lack of proper training results in overtreatment or undertreatment of the warts, which increases the likelihood of complications, including prolonged healing or infection.

When Surgery for HPV Becomes Necessary

While for many women topically applied treatments are all that's needed to eliminate genital warts, for some, HPV can be particularly stubborn. When this is the case, the CDC reports surgery may be necessary. The three basic methods are:

- Electrocautery. An electric current is used to burn away the warts.
- Laser therapy. A laser beam of high-intensity light vaporizes the warts.
- Excisional biopsy. Usually necessary only for large clusters of warts, this procedure surgically removes the tissue.

Since these procedures can be painful, treatment often requires anesthesia. In addition, the healing process can also be painful, and studies show all three surgeries may increase your risk of developing serious, chronic vulvar pain (see Chapter 5).

And, regardless of what type of surgery you choose, experts say it's vital that you return to your doctor for a follow-up check-up in about six months to confirm that no infection has developed and that all your warts have cleared.

Pregnancy and HVP Treatments

At least one type of genital wart, condylomata, can flare up during pregnancy, though no one is certain why. However, experts say never to use any medication from a previous infection, regardless of what that infection is, unless your doctor says it's okay, particularly while you are pregnant. Medications do have a shelf life, and problems associated with using an out-of-date drug can range from no results to toxic complications. But even more important, many otherwise safe medications are not safe to use during pregnancy. In the case of Aldara, no adequate studies have been done to support or condemn its use during this time. According to the new CDC treatment guidelines, however, you should avoid treatment with podophyllin and podofilox during pregnancy, and interferon may cause flulike symptoms when used during this time.

It is, however, important that warts be treated, particularly if they are large, since sometimes these growths can obstruct labor and facilitate the need for a cesarean section birth. Talk to your doctor about which treatments are safest for you and baby.

Toothpaste, Vaccines, and Cervical Cancer

Can something as common as toothpaste help protect you from cervical cancer? As odd as it sounds, the answer may one day be yes. New studies have shown that an ingredient commonly found in both toothpaste and shampoo—sodium dodecyl sulfate or SDS—appears to kill strains of HPV that are linked to cervical cancer. Further, only a low concentration is needed (about one-thousandth of what you normally find in a bottle of shampoo) kills the virus in the lab.

But before you start squirting Crest into your diaphragm, remember that studies are only preliminary. What's more, what often works in the lab doesn't pan out in real life. If, however, studies do continue to verify the effectiveness of SDS, expect a specially prepared product on the market around 2005.

Additionally, a number of clinical trials are underway for what is likely to be the first vaccine against cervical cancer. Currently under investigation by the National Cancer Institute, the shot is designed to protect against HPV 16, the strain responsible for up to 50 percent of all cases of cervical cancer, as well as anal cancer in both men and women. So far the NCI reports that the vaccine is safe. Now it is testing its effectiveness.

Treatment vs. No Treatment

Although there are a variety of ways in which to treat genital warts, do keep in mind that no treatment is also an option. When left alone, genital warts can go one of three directions: they can disappear, remain the same, or grow larger. As long as you are not in any significant pain, taking a wait-and-see attitude won't harm you. And since genital warts are generally not indicative of cervical cancer, avoiding treatment is not likely to increase your risk of any serious consequences. In fact, currently, there is virtually no evidence to show that removing the warts will affect the natural course of the disease or reduce transmission rates. Indeed, whether the warts are present or not, the virus still remains in your body and can easily be passed on.

It's also important to note that even the most dramatic of treatments, including surgery, won't guarantee that you will be wart free forever. For many women the growths come back, sometimes within months of treatment.

The point here is that if your warts are not causing you any discomfort and your Pap smear, and hopefully a DNA HPV test, show no signs of cervical cancer, then experts say it is perfectly okay to leave your warts alone. You should still remain vigilant about regular Pap smears and consider being tested twice a year.

Virus #2:
Herpes

When it began appearing on the social scene during the late 1960s and early 1970s, genital herpes rocked the very foundation of the sexual revolution. As the first widespread STD for which there was no cure, the idea that you could contract a lifelong illness from a single night of casual sex threw more than just a wet blanket on our collec-

---

AN EXPERT'S OPINION ON . . .

Vitamin A and HPV

Q: I've heard that certain vitamins can reduce the risk of genital warts and maybe even cure the ones you have. Is this true?

A: Certainly many believe that vitamins can increase your immunity to disease by helping to ensure that your immune system is supplied with all the nutrients necessary to run at peak performance. As to specific nutrients and their effect on HPV, studies presented at the 1999 Sixth Conference on Retro-viruses and Opportunistic Infections in Chicago noted that a *deficiency* of vitamin A was associated with an increased risk of precancerous cervical abnormalities, particularly when HPV was also present. Early animal studies also found an association between low levels of vitamin A and the development of premalignant lesions.

Although no one is certain if taking vitamin A when a deficiency does not exist will offer you any protection against HPV, many experts are looking at the possibility that this nutrient may have some protective effects, and future studies may one day show this to be true.

TREATMENT FOR TWO?

Q: I'm being treated for genital warts, but my doctor never mentioned if my partner should be treated or even examined. Isn't this unusual, and shouldn't my partner be treated to make certain I don't get the warts back?

A: Once you have HPV, it is with you for life. There is no such thing as being "reinfected." Having your warts removed means only that you are wart free, not free of HPV. The only reason your partner should be tested is if he too has warts and would like them analyzed and removed. In terms of your health, however, it's not going to make much difference either way. The CDC *does* suggest that your partner be checked for other types of STDs, such as gonorrhea or chlamydia, since warts can increase the risk of contracting these infections.

tive libido. It helped usher in what would turn out to be one of the most significant social changes of the century. The words *sex* and *safe* were paired together for all eternity, and our fantasies, and particularly our reality, would never be the same.

Today there are some half-million new cases of genital herpes diagnosed every year, and the CDC reports some 45 million folks are currently infected with this virus, up some 30 percent from the 1970s. Most of the infections are caused by just two strains of the herpes virus, HSV 1 and HSV 2. Both enter the body through tiny breaks in the skin or mucous membranes, causing a kind of nerve inflammation that results in painful, itchy lesions that travel nerve pathways and settle either in and around the genitals or on the lips of the mouth.

While in the past HSV 1 was thought to be confined to areas above the waist (causing primarily cold sores on the mouth) and HSV 2 was limited to below the waist (causing genital blisters, pain, and itching), since the 1990s the line between the two viruses has blurred significantly. This, say experts is due at least in part to the popularization of oral sex that resulted when couples began bypassing intercourse as a way of avoiding infection with HIV.

Unfortunately, you don't need intercourse to contract either form of herpes. Perform oral sex on a partner with genital herpes (HSV 2), and you can suddenly find yourself with that same infection in your mouth. Meanwhile, if a partner with oral herpes (HSV 1) performs oral sex on you, you can end up with a case of genital cold sores.

Complicating matters further, either HSV 1 or 2 can be spread by almost any skin-to-skin contact. If your partner, for example, touches his own genital lesions and then touches your V zone, the infection can be passed on. In addition, a condition known as viral shedding makes transmission possible, even if direct contact with the lesions does not occur. In this instance, infected cells are shed onto surrounding skin. Indeed, while reporting at the 1999 Thirteenth Meeting of the International Society for STD Research in Denver, Dr. Richard Dicarlo, associate professor of medicine at Louisiana State University School of Medicine, said "There is ample evidence that the majority of persons infected with HSV-2 will shed the virus periodically, even in the absence of clinical manifestations." According to Dr. Dicarlo, with sensitive testing, shedding was detected on approximately 30 percent of days, even when no symptoms were present.

What does that mean for you? If your skin touches your partner's genitals while the virus is shedding, you can contract herpes.

While condoms and spermicide can reduce some of your risks, because this virus can be present in the entire genital area (and not just where the lesions are visible), the amount of protection they offer can be minimal.

Herpes and Your Body: What to Look For

If everyone who contracted herpes had the characteristic lesions, the virus would be far easier to avoid. Many folks, however, have no symptoms, so neither they nor their partners know they are infected. But just because you don't see symptoms doesn't mean you are not contagious. According to the American Social Health Organization, one in five people with herpes are silent carriers, able to transmit the virus without having any visible signs.

For those who do exhibit symptoms, the CDC reports that the most common signs are clusters of small blisters filled with a yellow-tinged liquid, beginning anywhere from two to ten days after exposure. The blisters can develop anywhere within the V zone—the labia, clitoris, and vaginal opening, as well as the buttocks, thighs, anus, and navel. According to the American Medical Women's Association, the blisters can also appear on the inside of the vaginal wall as well as on the cervix.

Many women experience an intense itching and burning as the blisters develop and even some V zone pain. There may be a more copious vaginal discharge and extremely painful urination, which results when the acid content of the urine splashes onto the blisters. Up to 88 percent of women with genital herpes also experience a coexisting cervical infection (cervicitis). Sometimes herpes breakouts are also accompanied by fever, swollen glands (in the genital region), headache, and muscle aches, particularly during the first episode.

Once the blisters rupture, the yellow fluid leaks out onto the skin, forming a crust, which lasts anywhere from one to three weeks. Some of the pain and itching diminish at this point, but the general discomfort can last until the crust clears. In women, the duration of the outbreak is usually twenty days; for men, the healing time is slightly less, about sixteen days.

About 10 percent of herpes patients develop a form of meningitis, which occurs when the virus attacks the membrane surrounding the brain. When this is the case, recovery can take somewhat longer.

On the mouth, a herpes infection causes a similar type of blistering, followed by the same crusting over of the skin. The full course of this infection usually runs about ten days to two weeks. It's also important to note that because the eyes contain mucous membranes, similar to what is in the mouth and the V zone, touching an infected lesion and then rubbing your eyes could cause the infection to spread to this area as well. Herpes in the eyes can lead to blindness.

Women Beware: Herpes Is Your Disease!

Like many other STDs, it is far easier for a man to pass HSV to a woman than it is for a woman to pass it to a man. One reason, say experts, is that women have a larger surface area of genital skin that is vulnerable to transmission. Plus, a woman's genital skin is thinner and more fragile than a man's, meaning it may be easier for the virus to penetrate. For that reason, women are at greater risk. According to the most recent National Health and Nutrition Examination (NHANES) study, the rate of herpes among women is 26 percent, while in men it is just 18 percent. According to reports in the *Journal of the National Medical Association,* African American women are affected most of all, with some 60 percent of black women now diagnosed with the herpes virus.

Increasing the risks for all women is having sex with an infected partner during menstruation or having rough sex that results in injury to the genitals.

Other high-risk factors are frequent intercourse, multiple sex partners, increased duration of sex, and the presence of other sexually transmitted diseases. There is also evidence that illnesses that weaken the immune system (such as cancer or HIV) or drugs that suppress its action increase risks as well. Other contributing factors are poor diet, caffeine, hormonal fluctuations, or active cases of vaginitis, yeast infection, or genital warts.

Tests and Treatments

Providing you are experiencing the characteristic lesions and blisters, most gynecologists will be able to diagnose your herpes infection on site. Some, however, may elect to perform a tissue culture, a test that involves gently removing some cells from an active lesion or fluid from inside the blister, to be sent to a laboratory for analysis.

Once your herpes infection is confirmed, there are medications that can help. Specifically, several new antiviral compounds work well to significantly reduce symptoms as well as the duration of each episode.

One of the first of these medications to be marketed was the drug acyclovir, which is still quite popular. Available as a topical cream, an oral medication, or an intravenous drip, essentially it works by limiting the ability of the virus to duplicate itself, which reduces the duration of each episode.

Newer antiviral drugs include the medications valcyclovir and famcyclovir, but to date, there have been no head-to-head studies

AN EXPERT'S OPINION ON . . .

Long-Term Herpes Infections

Q: I've heard that herpes is a permanent infection—in the sense that it keeps coming back. But after experiencing recurrences for about three years, I am now herpes free for over two years. Is it possible my body overcame the infection?

A: The latest studies published in the July 1999 edition of the *Annals of Internal Medicine* suggest it may be possible. After following more than 600 herpes patients for four years, researchers from the University of Washington in Seattle found that the majority of those with chronic genital herpes did experience a decrease in frequency of symptoms over time.

Additionally, Dr. Craig G. Burkhart of the Medical College of Ohio reports in the journal *Infections in Medicine* that "patients generally begin to notice a significant reduction in recurrence rates of clinical lesions by the seventh year after infection." Regardless of whether you use any medication to suppress outbreaks, says Dr. Burkhart, the number of outbreaks you will experience will likely decrease over time.

Studies also show that while women generally have a lower rate of recurrence beginning as soon as the second year after infection, men have similar rates of infection in both year one and year two. The difference, say the researchers, may be linked to after-care: it appears that women are better than men at going back to the doctor for a follow-up exam.

It's also important to remember that up to 10 percent of all herpes patients have only one infection and never experience any recurrence.

comparing all three medications against one another. However, when compared to placebo, studies conducted at George Washington University found that oral famcyclovir administered within the first seventy-two hours after breakout did decrease the risk of subsequent outbreaks by a significant margin. According to at least one researcher who worked on the study, it's possible that taking famcyclovir very early on may help stem the tide of *all* future outbreaks.

A second study conducted at the University of Maches in Great Britain compared famcyclovir to acyclovir and found similar results. Their research showed that only one of twenty-four patients taking famcyclovir during the first herpes episode had a recurrence within six months. By comparison, twelve of sixty-three patients treated with acyclovir returned with additional lesions within that same time period.

And finally, studies conducted at East Carolina University in Greenville, and published in the *Journal of the American Medical Association,* found famcyclovir to be the clear winner again. Up to 80 percent of patients remained herpes free following treatments, as compared to just 22 percent who took a placebo.

On the horizon. Two brand-new drugs, which Canadian clinical trials have shown to be very effective in reducing the symptoms and duration of genital herpes, are now in development. The medications, called edoxudine and alphainterferon, may be available in the United States early in this century, along with a herpes vaccine that is also in development.

While antiviral treatments are generally administered only after an outbreak occurs, if you experience six or more in a year, any of these medications can be prescribed as a preventative, to be taken on a regular basis even if you have no active infection. In addition to helping curb breakouts, preventative treatment can also control viral shedding, where contagious herpes cells can be present on the skin with or without lesions.

When You Haven't Got Time for the Pain

Although the pain and itching associated with a herpes outbreak may prompt you to try an anesthetic cream or even a cortisone preparation, experts say this is not a good idea. The reason: they can keep the lesions moist, which can cause the infection to last longer. In addition, there is some evidence the corticosteroids may increase the risk of secondary infection, mainly by keeping the lesions from healing.

Since passing urine can be painful for women with herpes (the acid causes irritation) you may find relief by urinating standing up, usually in a shower stall. Another option is to urinate through a tube made by cutting the bottom from a small plastic or paper cup, slitting the side seam, and rolling the material into a tube about the width of a tampon.

In addition to coping with the active infection itself, whenever herpes lesions are present there is a concurrent risk that a secondary bacterial infection may develop. This can lead to more pain and increase the duration of your outbreak. However, experts say problems can sometimes be avoided by using a mild soap to keep the genitals clean and then thoroughly drying the area afterward. This is best done with a hair dryer set on cool rather than with a towel, which can spread the infection.

Herpes and Pregnancy

Today there is far less hysteria about herpes infections during pregnancy than in the past. Still, there remains cause for concern. While the virus won't cross the placenta—meaning you can't transmit herpes to your baby during pregnancy—some studies show that infections that occur during the first trimester increase the risk of miscarriage.

More commonly, however, the real threat to your baby comes at delivery, when passing on the virus is a very real danger. According to studies on some 7,000 pregnant women published in the *New England Journal of Medicine,* among those who acquired their infections shortly before labor, nearly half the babies born were infected during the birth. One in nine of those infants died, and an equal number suffered long-term neurological consequences. Also, studies conducted in 1998 at Massachusetts General Hospital in Boston revealed that infants born to mothers with an active herpes infection were at risk for localized skin and eye lesions, as well as central nervous system infections. Thus, the later in your pregnancy that herpes lesions appear—through either a recurrence or an initial infection— the more likely it is that your newborn will be affected.

To help reduce the risk of problems, many doctors now routinely schedule cesarean births for any women who have experienced even one herpes infection during pregnancy. Others, however, limit C-sections to only those who have an active infection *at the time of the birth.* While this is obviously a more conservative approach, you must remember that many herpes infections are contagious up to a week before symptoms appear, so you could have the virus present in your V zone and not even know it. Indeed, one small study found that thirty-nine out of fifty-six women who gave birth to herpes-infected babies showed no evidence of active lesions at the time of their delivery, yet the babies were born with herpes.

If you have had herpes in the past or even if you suspect you may be carrying a silent infection (if your partner, for example, experiences active lesions), be certain to mention this to your obstetrician. If you experience a breakout during pregnancy, also make sure your doctor knows about it, and do discuss the advantages that a cesarean birth can offer.

Virus #3:
Hepatitis B

If you're like most other folks, you probably don't associate your liver, or particularly liver *disease,* with sex. The truth is, however, that a sexually transmitted virus known as hepatitis B (HBV) heads straight for the liver, sometimes attacking with such vicious force that death can result. According to the Hepatitis B Foundation (see the Resources section) HBV is the leading cause of liver cancer, claiming some 5,000 American lives each year. More commonly, however, HBV results in chronic liver disease, and a highly contagious STD that can remain with you for life.

FOOD, SUN, AND HERPES

Q: I've heard that certain foods, such as chocolate and cola, can trigger a herpes outbreak, and also that the sun can increase the risk of an outbreak. If so, will avoiding these foods help keep a herpes infection from occurring?

A: Some experts believe that certain foods encourage herpes outbreaks, and yes, chocolate is one of those foods. The key ingredient is the amino acid arginine, which studies show appears to aggravate the virus if it's already present in your system. Other foods that contain high levels of arginine include grains, cereals, nuts, seeds, beer, and most soft drinks. Avoiding these items during times when your immune system is already compromised (if you are very tired, for example, or if you have a cold) may help stave off a breakout.

At the same time, the amino acid supplement lysine (500 to 1000 mg three times a day) has been shown to reduce the rate of viral replication. However, since this supplement can cause a serious rise in cholesterol levels, check with your doctor before trying this treatment.

Finally, for reasons no one clearly understands, the sun does appear to encourage a herpes breakout. While it won't increase your chances for contracting the infection initially, once the virus is in your system, studies show the sun may trigger an attack.

Are You at Risk for HBV?

There are three types of hepatitis, known as A, B, and C. Only the B type is generally associated with sexual transmission. Harbored in body fluids, such as semen, vaginal secretions, saliva, and blood, transmission occurs when tiny cuts or abrasions in your body allow entry of infected body fluids. While you can get hepatitis B in other ways—through tainted blood products, by sharing a toothbrush or a razor with an infected person, or by having your ears pierced, your body tattooed, or even your nails manicured with equipment that has not been properly sterilized—research shows that up to 60 percent of all cases *are* sexually transmitted. Currently, the CDC estimates that one in twenty Americans will contract HBV in their lifetime, and, say the experts, it is 100 times more contagious than HIV, the virus that causes AIDS.

The factors that can increase your risks include:

- Multiple sex partners
- A male partner who is having sex with another man
- Living in the same house with a chronic HBV carrier
- Using IV drugs

You are also considered at high risk if you have the bleeding disorder hemophilia, or if your parents were born in Southeast Asia, Africa, the Amazon Basin of South America, the Pacific Islands, or the Middle East.

The Symptoms: What You Need to Know

According to the Hepatitis B Foundation, among the most obvious and earliest signs of HBV is the development of mild flulike symptoms, including low-grade fever, headache, muscle aches, fatigue, loss of appetite, and sometimes nausea, vomiting, and diarrhea, usually beginning anywhere from ten days to two weeks after exposure. Because symptoms of the virus can come and go within a few weeks, many people believe it is the flu and don't even realize they have HBV. And for up to 90 percent of those who do contract the virus, it doesn't matter, because it clears from their body without any further consequences.

However, for about 15 percent of HBV patients, the Foundation reports, the virus becomes chronic, remaining in the body for life. Some people may experience regular symptoms, similar to those felt at the onset of the disease, but for many, the infection will be silent, at least for quite a number of years. But just because you don't look or feel sick doesn't mean you aren't. Indeed, chronic HBV causes a continual liver inflammation, one that eventually can lead to serious, even life-threatening liver disease. Warning signs often include a dark, foaming urine, a pale-colored stool, some abdominal pain, and a yellowing of the skin and particularly the whites of the eyes. About 1 percent of those who develop chronic HBV, reports the Foundation, go on to experience a deadly form of the disease known as acute fulminant hepatitis. When this is the case, often a liver transplant is the only hope for survival.

What's also important to remember, however, is that carriers of chronic hepatitis B also remain contagious throughout their life, able to transmit the virus at any time, even if they have no outward symptoms. This, in fact, is one of the reasons that the virus has spread to the extent that it has.

Protecting Yourself from HBV

As frightening as all this sounds, remember that only a small portion of those who contract HBV do develop the chronic form. What's more, for those who do, a variety of medications can help. The key, however, lies in getting a quick diagnosis, and there are a number of tests to ensure that you can.

According to the Hepatitis B Foundation, if you believe you have been exposed to HBV or think you are at high risk the following tests can help:

HBsAg (hepatitis B surface antigen). This is the outer surface of the hepatitis B virus, and it triggers the antibody response. A positive test result means you are infected with HBV and can pass it on to others.

Anti-HBs (antibody to hepatitis B antigen). The presence of antibodies in your system means you have been exposed to HBV in the past, but it successfully cleared from your body. A positive test result means you now have immunity to future infection from HBV. You won't get it again.

Anti-HBc (antibody to hepatitis B core). This test identifies either a past or present infection and is usually positive in chronic carriers of the disease. However, if the anti-HBs test is also positive, it means you are likely recovering from a recent bout with HBV and are not a carrier.

For those who are diagnosed as having the chronic form of HBV, the following additional tests are suggested:

"E" antigen: High levels mean you are highly infectious; low levels mean you are less likely to pass the virus on.

Liver function tests to assess your general state of health

AFP (alpha-feto protein): While high levels are normal in pregnancy, for everyone else they could signal liver cancer.

Ferritin: Because your liver stores iron, high iron content in the blood may mean that liver destruction is underway.

In addition, if you are diagnosed with chronic HBV, talk to your doctor about treatment with the following medications: Intron A, Roferon-A, Welferron, Epivir-HBV, and beta interferon.

In addition to testing for HBV, you can also protect your health with a highly effective HBV vaccine, in use in the United States for over ten years. According to the American Liver Foundation, to date, some 5 million Americans and 20 million men and women worldwide have already safely received this inoculation. Generally administered in three injections over the course of six months, it is routinely given to health care workers, including doctors, nurses, dentists, and hygienists.

In addition to offering you protection before you are exposed, this vaccine also works after the fact. Indeed, if you obtain your inoculation within fourteen days of being exposed to HBV, you may still escape infection.

If you decide to be vaccinated, you must be tested for the virus first. If you have a current infection (and remember that you might not have any symptoms) or if you have had the virus in the past, you don't need the vaccine and should not receive it.

Additionally, if you have been diagnosed with any autoimmune disease, including lupus, multiple sclerosis, scleroderma, or rheumatoid arthritis, talk to your specialist before getting the HBV vaccine.

Pregnancy and HBV

If you are exposed to HBV after you are pregnant, contact your obstetrician immediately. Just because you were exposed doesn't mean you have the virus—but you do need to be tested. If you show no signs of the virus, you should consider the vaccine to ensure that you don't contract HBV. Why is this important? Studies show that 90 percent of women who develop HBV during pregnancy pass the infection to their newborns during delivery. Because babies are essentially born without a developed immune system, they can't fight the infection and have anywhere from a 10 to 90 percent chance of developing a chronic form of the disease.

If you test positive for HBV, your doctor can schedule a cesarean birth, which will reduce transmission risks to your baby, who can also be vaccinated at birth for further protection.

TALKING POINTS: TESTING FOR HBV

Because HBV testing is not routine, even during an annual primary care physical, you must specifically talk to your doctor about being screened. If you have problems discussing your sex life with your physician, remember that HBV can be contracted outside the bedroom, so you can comfortably request testing without having to go into details about your intimate encounters. You can, for example, mention that you are concerned about the cleanliness of the shop where you have your nails done or that you have recently had your ears pierced and are concerned about health and safety. Of course it's always a better idea to be honest with your physician—and, more important, to find a doctor in whom you can confide. That said, if you need to break the ice about HBV testing, you can use these other methods of transmission to open dialogue with your doctor.

Virus #4:
HIV–AIDS

As recently as the 1990s, most of the world believed that HIV, the virus that causes AIDS, was of little concern to women. Indeed, when first reported in the United States in 1981, the majority of AIDS cases were confined to homosexual men, particularly those who also used intravenous (IV) drugs.

This is no longer true. While the homosexual population and IV drug users remain at increased risk, any man or woman who is sexually active is considered at risk as well. Sadly, vulnerability among women is increasing at an alarming rate. From 1985 to 1996 the number of reported AIDS cases in American women increased from 7 percent to a whopping 20 percent. As we begin a new century, the World Health Organization (WHO) estimates 13 million women around the globe will be diagnosed as HIV positive. Indeed, today infection with HIV is the third leading cause of death in women aged twenty-five to forty-four, and it is the leading cause of death among black women in this age group.

What may surprise—or even shock—you is that studies show that male-to-female transmission of HIV is the leading cause of the disease worldwide. According to the American Medical Women's Association, women are also at greater risk for contracting HIV than men. One reason is that semen, even from a healthy man, neutralizes the protective acids found naturally in the vagina. Thus, a simple act of ejaculatory intercourse naturally increases a woman's risk of infection. Moreover, studies show that a single ejaculate of semen from an HIV-positive man contains far more HIV cells than are found in the vaginal secretions of an HIV-infected woman.

This is of particular concern since some of the latest studies—research conducted by Dr. Julie Overbaugh of the Fred Hutchinson Cancer Center in Seattle, Washington, and published in the January 2000 issue of *Nature*—revealed that when the transmission of HIV from man to woman occurs, the woman is likely to be infected with *multiple* strains of the virus. When men contract the virus from women, the study showed usually only one strain is involved.

Why is this important? The more varied the strains of HIV, the harder it may be to find a drug that is capable of holding back the replication process.

HIV: Your Personal Risk Profile

HIV is a virus that is spread primarily through the transmission of body fluids, including blood, semen, vaginal secretions, and urine. It can also be passed from mother to child in the amniotic fluid (the liquid that surrounds the baby in the uterus) as well as in breast milk. Prior to 1985, many HIV infections were acquired when patients received blood transfusions tainted with the deadly virus. Today, however, that risk is almost nonexistent.

While IV drug use is still a major source of infection, the primary mode of transmission is vaginal or anal intercourse. If you have any open sores in your mouth, oral sex may increase your risk as well. You can contract HIV when, during intimate activity, small breaks or cuts in the mucous membranes of your V zone, including your vagina and anus, allow the body fluids of an infected partner to gain entry to your bloodstream. What can increase risks even further is a sexually transmitted disease.

According to researchers at the Northwestern University Medical School, infections such as herpes, HPV, chlamydia, and any genital ulcer disease allow HIV to more easily enter and infect the V zone cells that would normally be involved in fighting the virus. Additionally, new data from the CDC reveals that normal cells that line the cervix help to protect against HIV transmission. But when these cells are altered by infection with other STDs, not only is that protection lost, the damaged cells may actually encourage the transmission of HIV over and above what the normal transmission rate might be.

In addition, according to studies conducted by Dr. Joan Kreiss, a researcher at the University of Washington in Seattle, any form of vaginitis that reduces your levels of the "good" lactobacillus bacteria in your vagina may also increase your risk of contracting HIV. The reason, reports Dr. Kreiss, is that lactobacillus appears to produce chemicals that fight infection, mostly by controlling the growth of other bacteria in the vagina. When, however, lactobacillus levels plummet, as they do in vaginitis, the risk of acquiring any infection, including HIV, goes up. More specifically, without the protection lactobacillus offers, the male-to-female transmission of HIV occurs far more often. Currently new drugs are under investigation that could supply the vagina with live lactobacillus bacteria, thus acting as a barrier to HIV.

Until something is available, however, you must remain particularly vigilant about either avoiding sex or at the very least using a properly fitted latex condom if you suspect you may have vaginitis, and your partner's HIV status is in question.

Also important to note is that, although the rate of HIV transmission among lesbian couples is very low, studies show rates do increase if you have sex with an infected female partner during a time when either of you is menstruating. Adequate protection must be used during this time.

How HIV Affects Your Body

Regardless of how HIV gets into your system, once it does, it begins progressively to impair, then ultimately destroy, the powerful cells of the immune system, your body's defense against disease. Thus, HIV will leave you extremely vulnerable to a variety of opportunistic infections, diseases that by and large are caused by microbes and other organisms that normally would not affect a healthy person.

In addition, HIV also increases susceptibility to some of the major killer diseases of our time, including cancer. Eventually so many immune cells are impaired or destroyed by HIV that the body can no longer defend itself against any infections. When the number of HIV cells in the blood becomes high enough, virtually all immunity to disease is lost, and the diagnosis of AIDS, acquired immune deficiency disease, is made. When an AIDS patient succumbs to this disease, death is usually the result of quite ordinary illnesses, such as pneumonia, that the body simply cannot overcome.

Although these facts paint a grim picture of HIV, the news is not all bad. Today the diagnosis of HIV is not considered the hopeless situation it was just a few years ago. Although still considered a deadly infection, advances in treatment are helping women with HIV live longer, healthier, more satisfying lives. Indeed, new antiviral drugs that help reduce the spread of HIV in the body, combined with new medications to treat the infections associated with this disease, can often mean that a woman could delay the onset of full-blown AIDS for up to twenty or thirty years. In some instances, it may never develop at all.

Could You Have HIV? How to Tell

Once HIV enters your body, incubation takes place almost immediately. However, it can take weeks or even months before any signs of the disease appear. Indeed, even an HIV test has what is called a window of opportunity—a period of about six months following initial infection in which even those who have the virus can test negative. That's one reason that your doctor may suggest repeating a negative HIV test within six months, particularly if you know for sure that you have been exposed to the disease.

When early symptoms of HIV do appear, anywhere from a few weeks to a few months after infection, you are likely to experience what seems like a bout of the flu—with aches and pains, chills and fever, and sometimes a sore throat. Much like the flu virus, these early symptoms clear in about two weeks. And for many women, this brief episode will be the only sign of infection for ten years or more.

For some, however, there can be a wide range of health problems that appear from time to time. These can include nonspecific symptoms such as swollen lymph nodes (glands located in the neck, groin, and under the arms), a lack of energy, weight loss, unexplained fevers and night sweats, skin rashes, and regular bouts of diarrhea. Specific V zone health problems linked to HIV include vaginitis and particularly yeast infections, in either your vagina or your mouth. In fact, stubborn and recurring vaginal yeast infections are so common among women with HIV that if you have this problem, don't be surprised—or insulted—if your doctor suggests an AIDS test may be in order. Women who are HIV positive can also experience menstrual difficulties, including irregular bleeding, the lack of any menstrual cycle, or highly irregular periods.

In 1993 the CDC expanded its definition of health problems linked to HIV in women to include cervical cancer, recurring bacterial pneumonia, and tuberculosis.

As HIV continues to impair the immune system, many women

become increasingly susceptible to a variety of more serious and even life-threatening illness, such as cancer and pneumonia. In later stages many HIV patients experience unusual sores on the mouth or tongue, an increased incidence of cold sores, unexplained shortness of breath, a dry cough, numbness in hands or feet, and even some personality changes.

Overcoming Your Fears: Taking Your First HIV Test

There is no question that taking an HIV test can be a harrowing emotional experience. Indeed, it's not every day that we purposefully put ourselves in a situation that could change our lives in such a major way. And, in reality, a positive diagnosis of HIV is a life-changing experience. However, it doesn't have to be as negative an experience as you might think. Indeed, the earlier your HIV status is discovered, the greater the number of treatments available to help you and, the more likely you are to hold off the truly ravaging effects of this disease for an indefinite period of time.

The best way to ensure you always have the maximum advantage is to have not just one but *regular* HIV tests, particularly when you start a new sexual relationship and again six months later. You should also consider being tested any time you believe your partner is having sex outside your relationship.

The test, which can be done at home or at a lab, is painless and involves only a small amount of blood. Results can be had in a matter of days—and the relief it can provide is worth every second of anxiety you may feel about taking the test.

If You Are Diagnosed with HIV: What to Do

Regardless of whether your HIV test was done at home or in your doctor's office, it's important that you seek the care of an HIV specialist—someone who can begin immediately to treat you aggressively.

Currently, there are some fifteen HIV drugs available, and often they are prescribed in groups. Research shows that taking multiple drugs at the same time, in what is known as an "AIDS cocktail," appears to increase results over and above taking large doses of a single

HOME TEST VS. LAB TEST: HOW TO DECIDE

In an effort to help relieve some of the stigma—and a lot of the fear—about being tested for AIDS, during the 1990s the FDA approved several at-home test kits. Most involve pricking your finger and placing a small amount of blood on a specially prepared slide, which you then send to a laboratory for analysis. Because the test is completely anonymous, each testing kit is assigned a code number, which you then use to call the company and get your result. For many people, it is the fastest and easiest way to be tested. In terms of reliability, studies show it is as accurate as the test a doctor would offer.

However, what the home kit can't provide is one-on-one counseling. Although those who receive a positive test result are usually provided with a hot line number where they can talk to specially trained counselors, sometimes the shock of discovering they are HIV positive can keep some folks from proper follow-up care.

Most experts agree that the best place to have an HIV test is in your doctor's office, where you will be in a trusting environment with someone who knows your medical history and cares about your health and welfare. If, for whatever reason, this is not possible, certainly a home HIV test is better than no test at all. If, however, you have a positive result, do see your doctor right away for a second test. Although the home tests are accurate, they are not foolproof, and mistakes can be made.

medication. Among the most common AIDS "cocktails" are the drugs zidovudine (AZT), didanosine (ddI), saquinavir, ritonavir, nevirapine, and the newest, amprenavir.

Should you develop any opportunistic infections associated with HIV, including mycoplasma or fungus infections, a number of new medications are available to help here as well. Indeed, the buzz surrounding these new drugs is so encouraging that many experts believe that one day soon, HIV will be considered a chronic but highly manageable disease—one that reduces life expectancy by only a small margin.

You can also increase your chances for a longer and disease-free life by observing the basic guidelines of healthy living. Studies show that getting adequate rest, reducing stress wherever possible, eating lots of fruits and vegetables, reducing your intake of red meats and fatty foods, avoiding recreational drugs including tobacco, and making sure to meet your daily requirement of vitamins and minerals can all go a long way in helping your body to work better and more efficiently under all adverse conditions.

Pregnancy and HIV: Why You Should Be Tested

According to the American Medical Women's Association, a woman who is HIV positive has a one in three chance of transmitting the virus to her unborn baby. Transmission occurs when the virus crosses the placenta, the membrane that allows your baby to receive nourishment from your body.

Because it's possible to harbor HIV for many years without any obvious signs, it's not unreasonable for your doctor to suggest an HIV test. Indeed, the American College of Obstetrics and Gynecology is now calling for all pregnant women to be routinely screened for HIV, mainly because there are drugs available that can be taken during pregnancy to reduce the baby's risk of infection.

Because children's immune systems are not fully developed at birth, any child born with HIV does not have the same life expectancy as an HIV-positive adult. This is why prebirth treatment is so essential.

You should also know that HIV can be passed from mother to baby during delivery, and breast-feeding can also pass on the virus shortly after birth.

Because a baby has the mother's antibodies in his or her blood at the time of birth, all children born to HIV-positive mothers will test HIV positive as well until they are between fifteen and eighteen months old. If they still test positive after this age, then it is very likely they do have HIV. Children who are infected with HIV and show symptoms within the first year of life have a very poor prognosis.

A Final Word

While all of the viruses mentioned in this chapter can present you with some serious health challenges, it's important to remember that regardless of the disease, early diagnosis and treatment will go a long way in helping you avoid many of the more serious and life-threatening complications.

Indeed, as we embark on a new century, many important strides continue to be made in the treatment of many viruses, including the ones mentioned in this chapter. And while we still have no way to cure a virus, new medications are being put to the test almost daily, and many experts believe that before long, we will have drugs that can treat these infections as easily as an antibiotic cures a sore throat. In many instances, it is, in fact, the AIDS epidemic that is spurring on the development of new and better antiviral compounds, and many of the newest medications being used to treat AIDS may one day help researchers better understand how to treat all viruses, particularly those that are sexually transmitted.

More important, it is everyone's hope that more vaccines will become available to prevent viral transmission, so that no one ever again has to fear that the pleasures we get from sex will be too quickly circumvented with sickness and disease. Until that time, however, it's imperative that you continue to follow safe-sex guidelines whenever you have an intimate relationship:

- Always use a fresh, clean, new latex condom for every act of intercourse.
- If there is any realistic concern about your partner's health, ask him to be tested for the most common STDs, including HIV, prior to having intercourse. Until he is tested, make certain he uses a condom and that he puts it on himself.
- Let your partner remove his own condom after ejaculation, and don't allow his penis to lie near your vagina after the condom has been removed.
- Always wash your hands with soap and water (lathering for at least fifteen seconds) before inserting a diaphragm.

- Consider being tested for the most common STDs whenever you start a new intimate relationship.

Most important, see your doctor at the first sign of any sexually transmitted disease, and be tested for any infection to which you have been knowingly exposed. Your goal is to have safer sex, not fearful sex—and nothing removes fear as quickly and easily as the medical tests that can verify that both you and your partner are healthy.

CHAPTER NINE

V Zone Hygiene

Your New Guide to Intimate Care

For most women, personal hygiene is simply an extension of good grooming. We wouldn't think of going out with dirty hair or without bathing, so most of us reason that we should also be as diligent about our intimate personal care. Ready to aid and abet that line of thinking is an entire industry of personal care product manufacturers, ready, willing, and able to not only supply us with the products to do the job, but also encouraging reinforcement every step of the way. Indeed, you would be hard-pressed to glance at a fashion or beauty magazine without seeing at least *some* enticing advertisements for a variety of feminine hygiene products from douches to intimate deodorants, washes, sprays, and other products designed to make us look, feel, and smell as fresh as a bouquet.

While it remains true that V zone cleanliness is important, the level to which many women take the concept is, say experts, not only unnecessary but possibly harmful—increasing our risk of V zone infections, reducing our fertility, and maybe even predisposing us to cancer.

So what about looking and feeling, and most especially *being* clean *and* healthy? Isn't that important? It is. But before you decide what you really need, it's also important to understand a bit about how your V zone works to cleanse itself and the ways in which you can encourage that natural, healthy process.

Your V Zone Ecosystem: Mother Nature at Her Best

If you've ever questioned whether Mother Nature is really a woman, all one need do is examine the natural functioning of the female body. It's clear she has saved the best for herself. Indeed, inside each of us is a remarkable natural feminine ecosystem that works 24/7 to keep our V zone healthy and disease free.

Relying on a variety of natural secretions, including discharges, mucus, oil, and even sweat, the vagina continually works to cleanse itself, while maintaining an internal environment that inhibits the growth of a wide range of bacteria, including those that cause odor. Never is this system working harder than during the menstrual cycle, a time when menstrual blood joins in the cleansing process as well.

Because of that, your V zone needs very little in the way of special care. Indeed, daily cleansing with water and a mild soap is all most women ever need to maintain good vaginal hygiene.

Unfortunately, not all women see it quite this way. Partly because of popular culture and sometimes the result of personal or ethnic beliefs, many believe that unless specific measures are taken to cleanse the vagina—particularly douching—they'll end up with the V zone equivalent of body odor or greasy hair. In reality, however, the only ones who benefit from this line of thinking are the makers of intimate care products. For the women who use them, the result can be an alarming *increase* in V zone health problems, a correlation that studies show is becoming increasingly hard to ignore.

To Douche or Not to Douche: Know the Facts

Perhaps the single most studied feminine hygiene habit is douching, the act of using a pressurized spray to flood the V zone with any number of solutions, from homemade formulas of vinegar and water to commercial products in fruit flavors and flower scents. The idea here is to use both the pressure and the liquid to wash away potentially odor-causing micro-organisms and, if a commercial product is used, at the same time lay down a layer of scent or flavor to ensure we smell (or taste!) as sweet as can be.

Unfortunately, it doesn't always work quite this way. Indeed, in one important analysis, a study of more than thirty years of research published in the *American Journal of Public Health* in 1997, doctors discovered that douching once a week or more was associated with an alarming increase in pelvic inflammatory disease (PID), up some 73 percent over women who did not douche. Further, the more frequently a woman douched, the higher her risk of PID—even when the study controlled for potentially compounding factors, such as increased number of sex partners.

These findings were reinforced by the 1998 study published in the *Journal of Infectious Diseases,* already mentioned in Chapter 2. Here researchers from the University of Washington learned that women who douched regularly had a 50 percent greater risk of contracting bacterial vaginosis (BV), a leading cause of PID. The probable cause, say experts, is that the douche solution (even plain water) washes away the protective lactobacillus organisms that help protect the V zone from disease.

Overall, researchers report that the actual act of douching, rather than the douching liquid itself, is the real culprit. The force with which the liquid—any liquid—is sprayed into the V zone seems to speed the disease-causing pathogens from the vagina through the cervix and into the uterus and fallopian tubes, where they undoubtedly do the most harm.

Finally, studies published in both the *Journal of Obstetrics and Gynecology* and the *American Journal of Public Health* reported an alarming link between douching and ectopic pregnancy. Here, blockages in the fallopian tubes keep the fertilized egg from traveling to the uterus. The egg then begins growing in the tube, a condition that requires termination of the pregnancy and can even lead to a life-threatening tubal rupture for the mother. Indeed, the pooled results from five different case-controlled hospital studies showed that women who douched were 76 percent more likely to suffer an ectopic pregnancy, ostensibly the result of douching-related PID. More recently, studies on some 500 women, published in the *Journal of Obstetrics and*

MENSTRUAL ODORS
AND DOUCHING

Q: My boyfriend has a very sensitive nose and says he can detect a vaginal odor from me, usually around midcycle. Douching seems to help, and since I don't douche any other time of the month, I'm wondering if this once-a-month cleansing is okay.

A: While it's true that the less you douche the less likely you are to suffer any consequences, in your case it's the timing that's of particular concern. Studies show that douching at midcycle may be riskier than at other times of the month, increasing your odds of infection over and above what might normally occur. The reason, say experts, is that immediately after your monthly bleeding ceases, your cervical opening develops a small, sticky plug of mucus, which works to block the passage of many bacteria into the reproductive tract.

As you approach midcycle (about twelve to fourteen days after the start of your last period), that plug begins to thin and is washed away more easily, particularly if highly pressurized douche equipment is used. Once the mucus is gone, the gateway to your reproductive organs is open, and your risk of infection goes up.

As to the odor your boyfriend is smelling, it's possible he's picking up some kind of natural "fertility" scent, a smell that unconsciously is telling him you are fertile and one that many men find attractive. More likely, however, you may be passing a tiny amount of blood during ovulation (something that is quite common), which then sticks to your panties and gives off the odor. In this case, try wearing a minipad or panty liner for a day or two midmonth, and pay extra attention to washing the *outside* of your V zone with mild soap and water.

If your boyfriend insists the smell really is very obvious (it would probably smell a little odd to you as well), see your doctor. You could have an infection or even an ovarian cyst that flares during ovulation and contributes to the odor.

Gynecology, found that women who douched once a week or more had twice the risk of ectopic pregnancy over women who did not douche at all.

Douching and Your Fertility: The New Link

Since douching is linked to PID, which can reduce your chances of getting pregnant, it's easy to draw connecting lines between feminine hygiene and infertility. But the correlation goes a bit deeper than

---

AN EXPERT'S OPINION ON . . .

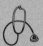

Douching and Cancer

Q: My sister was just diagnosed with cervical cancer, and her doctor told her that her constant obsession with douching may have played a role. Is this true? And will occasional douching have the same effect?

A: Since the 1930s, some researchers have suspected links between cervical cancer and douching, but for many years there was little in the way of concrete evidence. In 1997, however, a meta-analysis of dozens of medical papers published between 1965 and 1995 revealed there may be cause for concern. According to the research, conducted by the Department of Community Medicine at the Mount Sinai School of Medicine in New York City, frequent douching *was indeed* shown to have a moderate association with the risk of cervical cancer. Among those women who said they douched frequently—more than once a week—the risk was even higher, by some estimates up to 86 percent higher than for those women who did not douche at all. So while it may not be a major risk factor for cervical cancer, clearly evidence suggests douching may play *some* role, possibly by speeding the passage of organisms capable of harming cervical cells.

WARNING:
THE COCA-COLA DOUCHE

Q: I've heard that douching with either Coke or Pepsi right after intercourse can help you avoid pregnancy. Is this true—and is it safe?

A: The rumors surrounding this unusual use of soft drinks began because both beverages are highly acidic, and acid can harm sperm. In reality, however, not only won't these douches work as birth control (in fact, douching of any kind right after intercourse may push whatever sperm are lingering in the vagina up into the cervix and a lot closer to conception territory), their high sugar content can deposit so much glycogen in your vagina that it may significantly increase your risk of yeast infection. Experts say it won't work and it could cause you harm. Don't even think about it.

that. In a study of some 800 women, published in the *American Journal of Public Health,* as early as 1996 researchers from the National Institute of Environmental Health Sciences (NIEHS) found that douching decreased fertility by as much as 29 percent each month, with young women (aged twenty-five to twenty-nine) the most likely to suffer the consequences. Again, the more you douche, the greater is your risk of problems. What's more, researchers also found that what was used during the douching process seemed to make no difference. Indeed, even simply spraying the V zone with plain water seemed to have detrimental effects on fertility.

Experts theorize that the simple act of douching itself may alter the vaginal pH (acid level) in such a way as to hamper or even kill sperm. Another theory is that douching propels bacteria (particularly those that cause chlamydia) deeper into the reproductive system, which in turn, may prevent a healthy implantation.

Telling the Truth About Douches

Right about now you might be asking yourself, Why, if douching is so dangerous, are these products even sold? One reason is that the manufacturers—and even some doctors—continue to maintain that, when used as directed, these products *won't* cause you any harm. And, in fact, if you avoid douching during ovulation and limit their use during other times of the month, you may not experience any significant consequences.

Others, however, believe the real truth about douches remains locked inside a knot of bureaucratic red tape. More specifically, because these products are considered a cosmetic and not a drug, they are *not* subject to the same proof-of-safety studies as medicines. Manufacturers are *not* required to prove that douches are either safe or effective, and therein may lie the loophole that fosters their popularity.

However, the question surrounding the safety of douches may not be left to linger too much longer. Concerned over mounting evidence linking douches to health risks, the FDA is reportedly considering reclassifying these products as drugs, forcing a whole new burden of proof on product makers.

A Final Word: When Douching *Is* Necessary

From time to time you may find that your doctor actually "prescribes" a douche—sometimes made from a simple vinegar and water solution, other times from medications or antiseptic solutions such as Betadine. In most instances your physician is looking to get medication into the nooks and crannies of your V zone or simply trying to provide some relief from inflammation. In either case, it's certainly okay, and even necessary, to use these products. Do, however, make certain to either throw away douching equipment after your final treatment, or wash it thoroughly using soap and very hot water. This can help reduce your risk of reinfecting yourself if you do choose to douche for other reasons later.

Soaps, Washes, and Powders:
What to Avoid

One of the unique aspects of the V zone anatomy are the mucous membranes that line the inside of the vulva, particularly the vagina. Much like the membranes found inside the mouth as well as in the eyes, this tissue is extremely porous, meaning it has an absorption rate many times more powerful than the skin. In many instances, this can be a good thing—when, for example, you need to internalize a topical medication quickly, such as a progesterone cream. Other times, however, it may not be such a good thing—when, for example, a feminine hygiene product or even a soap contains questionable ingredients. Then the porous nature of your V zone could increase your risk of problems, particularly sensitivity reactions.

For most women, the majority of V zone product-related problems fall under the heading of contact dermatitis—a rash, irritation, or inflammation that results when one or more ingredients in a product comes in contact with your delicate V zone membranes, causing a sensitivity reaction. If you also happen to have another V zone inflammation occurring at the same time, such as a yeast infection or any other type of vaginitis, your risk of a sensitivity reaction is even greater.

Among the most common ingredients to cause such problems are perfumes and dyes, which can be found in everything from soaps and shower gels to deodorant sprays and even scented panty liners, toilet paper, sanitary pads, or laundry detergents. But the real problem here isn't always what you smell, or even what you see on the label. The reason? According to the FDA, many products that are labeled "unscented" do in fact contain traces of fragrance, sometimes enough to initiate a sensitivity reaction.

The same is true for those labeled "hypoallergenic." While in laboratory tests, these products are less likely to cause allergic problems, including contact dermatitis, it doesn't mean they are allergy free.

The point here is that if you are experiencing a V zone irritation, don't automatically dismiss seemingly benign personal care products, such as items labeled "unscented" or "hypoallergenic," as possible

SAFE SOAP: WHAT TO USE

While frequent baths (five times a week or more) may lead to V zone problems, it is still important to maintain intimate cleanliness. According to experts at the Center for Vulvar Diseases at the University of Michigan Medical Center, the best soaps for cleansing the V zone are Neutrogena, Basis, Pears (made in England), and castile soap with olive oil.

Experts caution never to scrub your V zone with a rough or harsh washcloth or loofah sponge, instead using only your hand for sudsing. Also be certain to dry your V zone thoroughly before getting dressed. If you have any infections, try using a hair dryer set to cool to facilitate drying the *outside* of your vulva. *Do not, under any circumstances, blow the air directly inside your vulva or vagina.* This could be extremely dangerous, with life-threatening complications, including the development of embolisms or blood clots.

culprits. Experts say the only way to know for certain if a product is causing your symptoms is to eliminate its use for two weeks or longer. If your irritation clears, try the product again—and then discontinue use at the first signs of trouble.

In addition, experts at the Center for Vulvar Diseases at the University of Michigan say to pay attention to the products you use to care for the items that come in contact with your V zone, such as the detergent used to wash your panties and panty hose, as well as your bathing suit or even your diaphragm. Remember that soap and detergent residues often remain, particularly on clothing, so don't overlook your intimate wardrobe as a potential cause of V zone irritation. To help cut down on potential problems, the center suggests washing intimate wear by hand, using a mild detergent such as Woolite or Ivory Flakes, and then rinse, rinse, RINSE! When possible, avoid the use of fabric softeners, particularly if they are scented, and don't rinse undies in perfumed water.

Finally, what you wear, in terms of the fabric of your V zone inti-

COULD IT BE A MAN ALLERGY?

Q: Is it possible to be allergic to a man? I just started having sex with a new partner, and each time we are together I develop an intense itching and burning in my vagina. It usually goes away in a few days but comes back right after sex with him again. He's using a lubricant and a condom, but I have no previous latex allergy. Could it be him?

A: While there is such a thing as a "man allergy" (some women have a sensitivity to a certain partner's sperm), most often it results in infertility and not the reaction you describe. What could be your problem, however, is your choice of lubricants. Is it scented or flavored, or does it contain dyes? These would be your most likely sources of trouble—but not the only ones. According to the Center for Vulvar Diseases, your best choices would include Astroglide, Lubrin, Moistur-el, Replens and K-Y Jelly. All are thought to be the least likely to cause problems.

The other factor to check is the condom itself. Besides the latex component, is it colored or does it contain talc? Both can be sources of irritation for women.

Finally, check with your new man about any soaps or fragrances he may be using in his P zone just prior to sex. This could also be the source of some irritation.

Finally, before you toss the man, you might also try a quick pre-sex shower for two, using the products you know don't cause you any problems.

mate wear, can also help reduce the risk of problems. Here, Center experts suggest that 100 percent cotton underwear, in white, is the least likely to cause problems. If you are prone to V zone infections or inflammations, doctors say refrain from wearing panty hose whenever possible, and avoid any undergarments that are made from synthetic materials such as nylon or Lycra spandex. These materials can retain body heat, which creates an environment that makes it easier for vaginitis to occur.

Bubble, Bubble, Toil and Trouble

Love ending your day in a warm, relaxing bubble bath? Many of us do, and experts say it is a great way to unwind. Do it too often, however, and don't be surprised if you end up with not only persistent V zone irritations but also recurring urinary tract infections. Studies conducted at the University of Colorado Health Sciences Center in Denver found that women who took five to six tub baths a week had a much higher rate of UTIs than women who bathed less frequently. In addition, nearly three-quarters of the women with the higher rate of UTIs also used moisturizing soaps in their bath. This study supported earlier research that found that for many women, the detergents used in bubble baths could also increase the risk of UTIs as well as vaginal inflammation. According to the FDA, it is the prolonged exposure to these ingredients—too many long, relaxing baths—that is the real source of the problem.

More recently, the FDA has expressed concern over National Toxicology Program (NTP) studies on DEA (diethanolamine) and DEA-related products—ingredients that act as emulsifiers or foaming agents in an alarming number of bath and shower gels as well as shampoos. The NTP found that when applied topically to rats and mice, DEA-related ingredients increased not only the risk of dermatological problems, including skin ulcers, but also cancer. Even more disturbing, in many instances, the female animals were far more affected than the males.

What makes these findings so relevant is that unlike other animal studies, where the testing ingredient is ingested, in this research the animals simply received dose-related topical applications. And while the results are not automatically transferred to humans, still the FDA is concerned enough about the findings to call for a more detailed internal review, with a keen eye toward a public health warning.

IS IT SAFE TO SPRAY?

Q: My husband is very odor conscious and so I've always used vaginal deodorant sprays. Now I'm wondering if there is a connection between these products and the constant vaginal burning I seem to be having these past few months. Is it possible the sprays are the reason?

A: Since most vaginal deodorant sprays contain fragrances, as well as chemicals used to propel the aerosol, they certainly have the potential to cause the symptoms you describe. The fact that you have been using them a long time without problems doesn't really matter, since sometimes a sensitivity can develop after long-term use. It's also possible that the product maker added something new to the formula—particularly in regard to the propellant, and that may be causing your symptoms.

Then again, it's possible you may be using the product too often, or spraying it directly on your skin. According to the FDA guidelines, feminine deodorant sprays should never be used inside the vulva, never applied to broken, irritated, or itching skin, and always be sprayed from a distance of at least eight inches from the skin.

Finally, don't spray your panties, sanitary pads, or tampons. This puts the chemicals in direct contact with your vaginal mucosa and, depending on the ingredients, they could be a significant health hazard.

You should also be aware that at least one study—research conducted at the Fred Hutchinson Cancer Research Center in Washington State—found that women who use vaginal sprays, particularly those with a powder ingredient, have as much as a 50 percent increased risk of ovarian cancer. Reporting in a 1997 issue of the *American Journal of Epidemiology*, the researchers say that the risks also increase with the length of time you use the sprays—long-term use yields the greatest risks.

If you are interested in avoiding DEA-related ingredients, the NPT says look for the following synonyms, which should be listed on your product label:

- Cocamide DEA
- Cocamide diethanolamine
- Coconut oil diethanolamine
- N, N-bis (hydroxy ethyl) coco amides
- N, N-bis (hydroxy ethyl) coco fatty amides

Feminine Hygiene and Ovarian Cancer: What You Need to Know

If you are like many other women, your bathing ritual somehow doesn't feel complete without a dusting of bath powder. This is particularly true in summer, when the powder can help absorb excess perspiration and make us feel cooler, drier, and more comfortable.

When, however, you use dusting powder in your V zone, that comfort may come at a high price—an increased risk of ovarian cancer.

Although once considered a hotly debated medical topic—not all doctors believed the dusting powder–cancer link was true—today most experts agree the correlations are hard to deny. Studies conducted by researchers from Brigham and Women's Hospital in Boston, Massachusetts, and published in the *International Journal of Cancer* as recently as 1999 concluded that the evidence linking the use of talc (either directly on the V zone or on sanitary napkins or tampons) with the incidence of some types of ovarian cancer is in fact so profound, it warrants far more formal public health warnings.

These findings back up earlier studies conducted at Yale University in 1997. Here, researchers found an equally overwhelming correlation between the use of talc and ovarian cancer. What's more, this study also revealed that while the frequency with which a woman used talc in the V zone didn't matter (once a week appeared to be as detrimental as five times a week), what did seem to make a difference was the duration of exposure and cancer risk—the longer a woman continued to use talc in her V zone, the greater her ovarian cancer risk.

AN EXPERT'S OPINION ON . . .

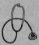

Dusting Powder vs. Baby Powder

Q: I know that it is dangerous to use dusting powder near the vagina, but I'm wondering if the same warnings hold true for baby powder. Don't mothers regularly use this on baby girls' genitals, so shouldn't it be safe for grownups?

A: In studies conducted at the College of Physicians and Surgeons at Columbia University in New York City, Dr. Carolyn Westoff analyzed ovarian tissue from twenty-four women whose ovaries were removed for reasons other than cancer. Upon analysis, talc was found in the tissue of all twenty-four women. Interestingly, however, only twelve of the women reported using any talcum powder as adults. This led researchers to conclude that widespread exposure to talc during the diapering process could contribute to the presence of talc in ovarian tissue as an adult.

This information, combined with studies showing that many babies suffer severe health consequences after inhaling talcum powder during diapering—some children have even died—has led many mothers to stop powdering their babies.

Also worth considering is that usually perfumes and dyes added to adult dusting powders can make them doubly treacherous for V zone use. However, if the powder component is talc, the most common form of powder, both baby and adult products carry the same risks.

In addition to dusting powder and talc, you should also be aware that your cancer risks may increase via the talc used in some condoms.

If you're absolutely hooked on dusting powder, you might want to seek out products that use cornstarch rather than talc as the basis for the powder. At least one report, a research paper issued by the American Health Foundation, says there is no evidence that the use of cornstarch-based powders in the genital area have any adverse effects. Although they do point out that the number of studies on cornstarch and ovarian cancer is small, the real point, according to authors John Whysner, M.D., Melissa Mohan, and Gary Williams, M.D., is that the very nature of the chemical construction of cornstarch makes it nearly impossible to be linked to ovarian cancer. Indeed, since cornstarch is used in foods and easily broken down by the body, at least theoretically, it should pose no significant health risk.

Silicone: Breast Implants May Be the Least of Your Worries

If you are one of millions of women who would not put silicone in your breast, why are you putting it in your bathwater? What's that? You didn't know you were?

The truth is that silicone and its many derivatives are found in dozens of bath products and an increasing variety of skin care and cosmetic products of all kinds.

Often concealed in preparations under terms like "dry oil" (and a top cosmetic manufacturer who uses that very term once confided to me confidentially that if they used the word *silicone* in products ads, they feared no one would buy it!), silicones can also be listed as a lubricant or more commonly under derivative names such as simethicone, dimethicone, trimethicone, disiloxane, or terracyclosiloxane. A quick look in the personal care aisle of your local supermarket or drugstore should tell you just how widespread the use of this ingredient has become, particularly during the late 1990s. Perhaps, not coincidentally, silicone started showing up a lot more often in personal care products right around the time the FDA banned its use in breast implants.

So what's the problem with silicones? To be fair, early studies linking this chemical to a variety of autoimmune diseases such as lupus continue to be challenged. Indeed, new studies released as recently as the end of 1999 concluded that there is in fact no link at all. On the other hand, we cannot ignore that, despite safety claims, breast implant manufacturers have been forced to pay a settlement to thousands of women who have become ill from what they believe are diseases related to their silicone breast implants. Nor should we ignore the fact that not only does the FDA refuse to permit the use of silicone breast implants, it has also refused to approve the use of liquid silicone injections for the medical treatment of wrinkles. What's more, the FDA is prohibiting doctors from using or promoting the use of these injections.

Certainly there is no direct published evidence linking the use of silicones in any bath or cosmetic products to any suggestion of illness. Still, it's important to note that unlike what was required of silicone injections, manufacturers that use silicone in their cosmetic or personal care products are under no obligation to do safety studies or publish the results of any studies they may conduct on their own. Moreover, the FDA cannot require companies to do safety testing of these products prior to marketing. The FDA also has no power to require manufacturers to file data on their ingredients, or to report consumer complaints or injuries that occur as a result of those ingredients. Indeed, all recalls of cosmetic products are in fact completely voluntary. If the FDA believes a product is hazardous to public health, it must first prove in a court of law that the ingredient in question is injurious to users.

The point here is that if all of the information on silicone has convinced you never to put a silicone implant in your breast, then you may want to think about using products containing large amounts of silicone anywhere delicate mucous membranes can more easily absorb product ingredients, including not only the V zone but also the eyes.

Safe and Healthy Menstrual Protection

For many years the primary concern over menstrual protection products was the link between toxic shock syndrome (TSS) and tampons. This rare but potentially fatal disease results when bacterial toxins (most often streptococci and staphylococci), many of which reside in

AN EXPERT'S OPINION ON . . .

The Microbiology of Lingerie

Q: I've been reading a lot about these antimicrobial products such as cutting boards and toys. Now I hear they are making underwear treated with this stuff, and I'm wondering whether it is safe to wear so close to the vagina.

A: If you're talking about panties that are treated with the antimicrobial compound known as triclosan (it's also found in many personal care products including deodorant soaps, underarm deodorants, and shower gels), then yes, they are likely safe. In fact, according to Dr. H. N. Bhargava, of the Massachusetts College of Pharmacy and Allied Health Sciences in Boston, triclosan has only rarely been associated with any skin irritations or sensitivity reactions when used in a variety of products. According to his research, published in the *American Journal of Infection Control* in 1996, triclosan is not a toxin, even when ingested orally, and it appears to have no carcinogenic properties.

That said, keep in mind that it's possible to have an adverse reaction to virtually *any* product, so if you try the panties and develop any symptoms (including redness or itching), don't wear them.

the vagina in normally small amounts, begin growing out of control. As they do, a poison is produced (called toxic shock toxin) that makes its way into the bloodstream, causing body-wide illness and the symptoms we know as TSS. The link between TSS and tampons: When left in the body for more than four hours, tampons can provide a convenient place for the bacteria to grow. Indeed, research conducted by the CDC indicated that high-absorption tampons—the kind that many women use for overnight protection—were the most likely to increase the risk of TSS. In addition, a few specific tampon designs, most notably the ones sold under the name brand Rely, as well as certain high-absorbency materials, were also found to play a role.

To help reduce the risk of TSS, the sale of these products was banned in the United States. To avoid problems when you are traveling out of the country, experts suggest you either carry your own brand of tampons from home or purchase only those brands that are also available in the United States.

To further decrease your risk of TSS, look for tampons that have the lowest absorbency possible to handle your menstrual flow. Currently, the FDA requires tampon manufacturers to state absorbency levels on the package using the following generic terms:

Junior—least absorbent (6 grams of fluid or under)
Regular—moderate absorption (6 to 9 grams)
Super—greater than normal absorption (9 to 12 grams)
Super-plus—the highest absorption rate available (12 to 15 grams)

Remember that the above terms always refer to absorbency and not size and the definition remains the same from brand to brand.

Toxic Shock Syndrome

Today the FDA requires that all tampons sold in the United States carry a TSS warning as well as a brief description of symptoms. In addition, the American Institute for Preventive Health suggests you pay close attention to the following warning signs, usually appearing just before or right after your period ends:

- Mild cases of TSS are characterized by a sunburn-like red rash, often on the soles of the feet and palms of the hands, along with a fever that is usually over 102 degrees.
- You may also experience a sore throat, body aches, vomiting, and diarrhea.
- In severe cases of TSS you may experience low blood pressure, as well as kidney, heart, and liver abnormalities and blood clotting malfunctions.

If you do experience any of these symptoms, particularly during or right after your period, remove any tampons immediately, and call your doctor right away. Treatment for TSS always requires hospital care—potent antibiotic therapy to combat the infection.

Because TSS recurs up to 30 percent of the time, particularly in menstruating women, if you have had this infection in the past, it's probably a good idea to avoid tampon use.

Protect Yourself!

While FDA measures have helped decrease the risk of TSS by a significant margin (in 1997 there were only 5 confirmed cases of menstrual-related TSS, as compared to 814 in 1990), many experts believe women must remain diligent in their efforts to avoid this disease.

Among the best ways to protect yourself is never to leave a tampon in your vagina for more than four hours. So unless you plan on getting up in the middle of the night to change, you should restrict tampon use to daytime only. At night, many experts still consider a pad to be the safest alternative.

You should also be certain to wash your hands with soap and hot water (lathering for at least 20 seconds before rinsing) before removing or inserting a tampon. This will reduce the risk of transferring bacteria into your vagina.

In addition, never insert two tampons into your vagina, no matter how small they are. Not only does this defeat the purpose of lower-absorbency products, you also run the risk of forgetting about the second one. Indeed, many doctors report that they often find old tampons inside women during a gynecological exam, sometimes pushed very far up as a result of trying to double up on protection.

Little White Lies? A New Sanitary Protection Health Debate

Could remnants of the same lethal chemical used in the Vietnam War—Agent Orange—be lurking in your tampons and sanitary napkins? That's the questions that became the eye of yet another sanitary protection storm.

The chemical in question is dioxin, a powerful pesticide that is a

AN EXPERT'S OPINION ON . . .

Cotton Tampons and TSS

Q: I've heard that all cotton tampons are healthier than the synthetic blends, particularly in regard to toxic shock syndrome. Is this true, and if so, would all cotton pads also be generally safer to use than the synthetic blends?

A: The first all-cotton tampons were tested in 1994 by independent New York University researchers Dr. Phillip Tierno and Bruce Hanna. According to their findings, synthetic materials used in sanitary protection products do amplify the production of certain TSS-causing toxins, while the cotton products do not. "The synthetic tampons are more absorbent than the cotton [and that] leaves behind a concentration of proteins that the bacteria use to manufacture the toxins found in TSS," says Dr. Tierno. Although side-by-side comparisons have not been done, it seems as if the all-cotton tampons may be safer in this regard.

Sanitary pads have no link to TSS. However, many believe that other factors associated with synthetic materials used in pads make them less appealing than the all-cotton varieties.

For information on where to purchase all-cotton (and even some organically grown cotton) products, see "Resources for Better Health" at the end of this book.

by-product of the chlorine bleaching process used in the manufacture of a number of paper and rayon products, including not only things like coffee filters, toilet paper, and disposable diapers but also commercially made tampons and sanitary napkins.

Classified as a major carcinogen (some experts have called it one of the most toxic substances ever created by humans), ongoing studies continue to show that dioxin may have a variety of damaging health effects, including the disruption of the hormonal and endocrine systems. In at least one study involving rhesus monkeys, exposure to dioxin resulted in an increased incidence of endometriosis, a painful immune-related menstrual disorder that is also a leading cause of infertility.

Because a number of different manufacturing processes continually cause dioxin residues to leach into the air, water, and soil throughout much of the United States, most of us are exposed to small amounts of this chemical every day. And since dioxin residues can also be found on other products, such as disposable diapers and coffee filters, many believe that even if dioxin residues are present on sanitary products (and not everyone agrees that it is) women who use these products would be at no greater risk for health concerns than anyone else in the world.

But that line of thinking takes us only so far. Enter the vaginal mucosa, and everything changes. "The vaginal mucosa is extremely absorbent, and no amount of this chemical is considered safe," says Dr. Tierno, the New York University Medical Center researcher who was among the first to study links between tampons and TSS. "Virtually anything you place on this tissue gets absorbed."

As you read earlier, the mucous membranes lining your V zone are extremely porous, meaning they rapidly absorb almost anything with which they come in contact—including dioxin residues. According to published reports, Peter deFur, a physiologist consultant who has worked for the Center for Environmental Studies at Virginia Commonwealth University in Richmond, Virginia, believes that the vaginal mucus, once exposed to dioxin, would have "near 100 percent absorption of the chemical. It crosses membranes, it is taken up, transported and stored," he recently stated in an exclusive MSNBC report.

Once inside a woman's body, dioxin accumulates in fatty tissue. "It can be measured 20 to 30 years after exposure because the amounts remain in your system," says Steve Stellman, a cancer researcher with the American Health Foundation in New York.

For that reason, some environmentalists point out that the twenty-four hour-a-day direct tissue contact with tampons for up to five days every month, and even the more limited contact made by sanitary pads, could cause women to absorb an excessive amount of dioxin, even if the levels in the products test out as relatively low.

When paired with other sources of dioxin contamination—remember that it's found in water, air, soil, and other paper products—many believe the amount found in the sanitary products may push women over the edge in terms of what is considered a safe and acceptable exposure limit.

Is the Fox Guarding the Hen House?

According to those who defend the safety of these products, including such manufacturers as Tambrands, Playtex, and Johnson and Johnson, if there is any residue, it is so small that it can't possibly cause us any harm. And they say that safety studies they have conducted show that this is precisely the case. The FDA has long backed up their point of view, repeatedly stating that they believe that all tampons and sanitary pads are safe and pose no significant health risks to women.

Still, despite a barrage of public reassurances, reports began surfacing charging that a congressional subcommittee uncovered memos wherein FDA scientists themselves admitted that not only were there no levels of dioxin considered to be safe, but that at least some tampons contain levels that are quite high. As a result of that report, the subcommittee chairman, the late congressman Ted Weiss, accused the FDA of purposefully downplaying the dangers to women by ignoring the findings of its own scientific committee.

It was only in reports that surfaced sometime later that FDA officials admitted never having tested the products themselves—they based their decisions on outside studies. Although the testing was in fact conducted by independent laboratories, critics were quick to point out the facilities were hired and paid for by product manufacturers.

Picking up the gauntlet in 1997 New York congresswoman Carolyn Maloney introduced into the Congress a bill for the nation's first "Tampon Health and Safety Research Act"—legislation designed to force the FDA to conduct its own independent studies of dioxin levels in tampons and a variety of other factors linking those products to health risks in women. Although the bill never made it out of committee, Congresswoman Maloney continues to reintroduce it each session. More important, she has opened the issue for wider and more studious debate.

A Kinder, Gentler Tampon? You Decide

In its most recent declaration on the subject of tampons and dioxin, issued in July 1999, the FDA continues to believe these products are safe. In a written statement, it says, "While at one time bleaching the wood pulp [used in making the fiber for the tampons] was a potential source of trace amounts of dioxin in tampons, that bleaching method is no longer used. Rayon material used in U.S. tampons is now produced using elemental chlorine-free or totally chlorine-free bleaching processes."

So does that mean they are safe now—but weren't before, when they told us they were? That is precisely the kind of ambiguous message that has continued to fuel the debate. In recent correspondence to the FDA, Congresswoman Maloney wrote that there is no evidence on which to base statements that tampons are virtually dioxin free, particularly since the new bleaching processes the FDA makes reference to do in fact release this chemical. Further, in letters to her senatorial colleagues about dioxin, Maloney wrote, "Exposure to this chemical has been linked to cancer, immune system suppression, pelvic inflammatory disease, and infertility, and has also been linked with increased risk for endometriosis. Men, women, and children are exposed to dioxin through the air and the water. It makes no sense for women to have an additional exposure through tampon use."

The Protection Alternatives

Since it is doubtful that any concrete answers on these issues will surface at any time soon, most of us will be left on our own to decide whether the convenience and ease of use of these products is worth any potential health price we might pay. For most of us, the answer will lie in moderation of use, at least until further research verifies that these products are indeed safe.

Another option is to explore several new types of sanitary protection products. Among the newest and more popular substitutes for pads and tampons are these (see "Resources for Better Health" for information on where to buy).

Menstrual cups: Small plastic or rubber collection devices that are inserted into the V zone much like a diaphragm. They are left in place for about 12 hours, where they collect the menstrual flow. Since they keep the blood from exposure to the air, there is virtually no menstrual odor. On the downside, some experts believe that certain types of menstrual cups at least theoretically hold a TSS risk equal to that of tampons. There are, however, no reported cases to date. Currently there are two types of menstrual cups available. One, called "The Keeper," which is reusable, costs about $35, and is said to last about ten years. The other, called "Instead," is a disposable soft plastic cup that costs about the same as tampons.

Padettes: A small pad-like product that is placed just inside the lips of the vagina, with the flaps of the labia holding it in place. Unlike a tampon, it does not go deep within the V zone. And unlike a traditional pad, there is less risk of dripping or shifting. Padettes are not, however, designed to be used alone, particularly on heavy-flow days. But when they *are* paired with a light-absorbency tampon, they can increase your protection without increasing your risk of TSS.

Reusable cloth napkins: Sanitary pads made of cloth that are washed and reused after every cycle. Usually made of 100 percent cotton (sometimes organically grown), they can virtually eliminate all risk of chemical contaminants providing they are properly cleansed. If washing dirty diapers by hand is not something you relish, these pads are not for you.

A Final Word:
Good Health Without Fear

Obviously, much of what you have read in this chapter has an ominous or maybe even a fearful tone. I can assure you, however, that this information was not included in this book to frighten you. It was meant to raise your awareness—not so much about what can harm you but about how, by making a few wise choices, you can protect your V zone health and avoid many future problems. I hope you will view this chapter not as a strict list of don'ts but rather as a cautious road map, one that can be used to help you sort through your intimate care options and find the treatments, products, and methods that are most beneficial to you.

Most experts agree that good health is often a matter of making choices: reducing risks in one area allows you to take a few liberties in other areas.

In light of that, I hope you use the information in this chapter to balance your V zone care. By combining what you learned here with your personal and family health history, I believe you will be better able to make the most intelligent choices for your life and your lifestyle.

RESOURCES FOR
BETTER HEALTH

American Foundation for Urologic Disease
1128 North Charles Street
Baltimore, MD 21201
410-468-1800
www.afud.org
email: *admin@afud.org*

American Liver Foundation
75 Maiden Lane, Suite 603
New York, NY 10038
800-465-4837
www.liverfoundation.org
email: *webmail@liverfoundation.org*

American Social Health Association
P.O. Box 13827
Research Triangle Park, NC 27709
919-361-8400
www.ashastd.org

American Society for Reproductive Medicine
1209 Montgomery Highway
Birmingham, AL 35216
205-978-5000
www.asrm.org
email: *asrm@asrm.org*

Center for Vulvar Disease
Obstetrics and Gynecology Department
University of Michigan
1500 E. Medical Center Drive
Taubman Center, Reception E
Box 0384
Ann Arbor, MI 48109
734-763-6295

Centers for Disease Control and Prevention
National Center for HIV, STD, and TB Prevention
1600 Clifton Road
Atlanta, GA 30333
800-311-3435
404-639-3311
www.cdc.gov

Fibromyalgia Network
P.O. Box 31750
Tucson, AZ 85751
800-853-2929
www.fmnetnews.com

Glad Rags (all-cotton cloth menstrual pads)
Keepers! Inc.
P.O. Box 12648
Portland, OR 97212
800-799-4523
503-282-0436
www.gladrags.com

Infectious Diseases Society of America
99 Canal Center Plaza, Suite 210
Alexandria, VA 22314
703-299-0200
www.idsociety.org
email: *info&idsociety.org*

Interstitial Cystitis Association
51 Monroe Street, Suite 1402
Rockville, MD 20850
800-435-7422
301-610-5300
www.ichelp.org

Low Oxalate Diet Book
General Clinical Research Center (H203)
University of California at San Diego
Medical Center University Hospital
225 Dickensen Street
San Diego, CA 92103
(Books are $5.00 each; checks payable to Regents of University of California)

National Black Women's Health Project (NBWHP)
600 Pennsylvania Avenue, SE, Suite 310
Washington, DC 20003
202-543-9311

National Center for Complementary and Alternative
    Medicine Clearinghouse
National Institutes of Health
P.O. Box 8218
Silver Spring, MD 20907-8218
888-644-6226
nccam.nih.gov
email: *nccamc@altmedinfo.org*

National Herpes Hotline
800-230-6039 (for written information)
919-361-8488 (for counseling)

National Kidney and Urologic Disease Information Clearinghouse
3 Information Way
Bethesda, MD 20892
301-654-4415
www.niddk.nih.gov
email: *dk_ocpl@extra.niddk.nih.gov*

National Kidney Foundation
Dept. UTI
30 East 33rd Street
New York, NY 10016
800-622-9010
212-889-2210

National STD and AIDS Hotline
800-227-8922

National Vulvodynia Association
P.O. Box 4491
Silver Spring, MD 20914
301-299-0775
www.nva.org

Planned Parenthood Federation of America
810 Seventh Avenue
New York, NY 10019
212-541-7800
www.plannedparenthood.org or *www.ppfa.org*
email: *communcations@ppfa.org*

Ragtime (all-cotton cloth menstrual pads)
3565 Clayton Road, #A
Concord, CA 94519
925-686-0366

Vulvar Pain Foundation
P.O. Drawer 177
Graham, NC 27253
910-226-0704
www.vulvarpainfoundation.org

On the Internet

Selected Sites of Excellence for Women's Health

American College of Obstetrics and Gynecology
www.acog.com

American Medical Women's Association (AMWA)
www.amwa-doc.org

HealthScout Network
www.healthscout.com

Journal of American Medical Association Women's Health Information Center
www.ama-assn.org/special/womh/womh.htm

Mayo Clinic Women's Health Center
www.mayohealth.org/mayo/common/htm/womenpg.htm

Medscape
www.medscape.com

National Women's Health Information Center
www.4women.org

OBGYN.net
www.obgyn.net/medical.asp

Physicians' Desk Reference
www.pdr.net

S.P.O.T. The Tampon Health Web site
www.critpath.org/~tracy/spot.html

Vulvodynia.com (Dr. Howard I. Glazer's Web site)
www.vulvodynia.com

Wellness Web Women's Health Center
www.wellweb.com/women/women.htm

Centers of Excellence
in Women's Health

National Women's Health Information Center/Office on Women's Health
U.S. Department of Health and Human Services
200 Independence Avenue, SW, Room 730B
Washington, DC 20201
800-994-9662
www.4woman.gov/coe

The Centers of Excellence in Women's Health across the nation are dedicated to providing state-of-the-art diagnostic and treatment regimens for women. To find the Center of Excellence in your area, call the toll-free information line or visit the Web site.

Complete bibliographical information, including references to all medical and research papers used in the preparation of this book, can be found online at *www.theVzone.net.*

INDEX